Principles in Health Economics and Policy

Principles in Health Economics and Policy

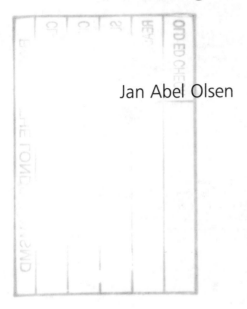

Jan Abel Olsen

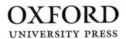

OXFORD
UNIVERSITY PRESS

OXFORD
UNIVERSITY PRESS

Great Clarendon Street, Oxford OX2 6DP

Oxford University Press is a department of the University of Oxford.
It furthers the University's objective of excellence in research, scholarship,
and education by publishing worldwide in

Oxford New York

Auckland Cape Town Dar es Salaam Hong Kong Karachi
Kuala Lumpur Madrid Melbourne Mexico City Nairobi
New Delhi Shanghai Taipei Toronto

With offices in

Argentina Austria Brazil Chile Czech Republic France Greece
Guatemala Hungary Italy Japan Poland Portugal Singapore
South Korea Switzerland Thailand Turkey Ukraine Vietnam

Oxford is a registered trade mark of Oxford University Press
in the UK and in certain other countries

Published in the United States
by Oxford University Press Inc., New York

© Oxford University Press, 2009

British Library Cataloguing in Publication Data
Data available

Library of Congress Cataloging-in-Publication Data
Data available

Typeset by Cepha Imaging Private Ltd., Bangalore, India
Printed in Great Britain by the MPG Books Group, Bodmin and King's Lynn

ISBN 978–0–19–923781–4

10 9 8 7 6 5 4 3 2 1

Whilst every effort has been made to ensure that the contents of this book are as complete, accurate
and up-to-date as possible at the date of writing, Oxford University Press is not able to give any
guarantee or assurance that such is the case. Readers are urged to take appropriately qualified medical
advice in all cases. The information in this book is intended to be useful to the general reader, but
should not be used as a means of self-diagnosis or for the prescription of medication.

Preface

This book is based on the view that there are four principal questions facing health policy makers in all countries. These four questions are universal in that they are equally relevant no matter how much money a country spends on its health services, and no matter the political system. The questions are recurrent in that they tend to pop up constantly when health policy reforms are being discussed. The structure of this book reflects the following logical order of these questions:

1) How should society intervene in the *determinants* that affect health?

Needs for health care depend on how our health is being affected by the physical and social environment as well as by our health related lifestyle. There are various ways in which the health affecting circumstances that surround us can be improved and healthy choices can be encouraged. To which extent should society intervene?

2) How should health care be *financed*?

The more needs for health care, the more money is required to finance it. Revenues can be raised through: i) patient payments ('out of pocket' at the point of delivery), ii) taxation (and social insurance), and iii) private health insurance. Rarely would we find that a country has chosen only one of the three sources, most often we find a combination of at least two. For which reasons would we prefer one source of financing over the other?

3) How should health care providers be *paid*?

Once revenues have been collected, there are various ways in which to pay providers of care. The key issue is whether it should be activity based or not. Hospitals may receive fixed annual budgets, or they can be reimbursed depending on how many patients have been admitted and what types of care have been provided. Primary doctors can be salaried, or remunerated depending on their number of patients and what services they provide. Why, and to what extent, should payments be activity based?

4) **How should alternative health care programmes be *evaluated* when setting priorities?**

Once revenues are raised and providers are paid, resources are allocated to competing health care programmes. If you believe that health care should be distributed on the same principle as ordinary market goods, resources would simply be allocated to those services that patients are willing and able to pay far. However, if you believe that health care should be distributed depending on people's needs, you must evaluate the competing alternatives in order to find where they improve the most health. Which methodologies are appropriate for assessing the degree to which new treatment programmes are efficient and equitable?

A closer look at these questions makes it quite evident that the answer you give to 4) would influence your answer to 2), in that *if* you think health care should be distributed according to health needs, then you cannot hold that all health care should be financed in a way that is dependent on ability to pay such as patient payment or private insurance.

Clearly, there are no universally correct answers to these questions. The answers depend on the objectives of the health service, and these objectives are normative in that they reflect value judgements. Interestingly though, most health policy objectives can be understood as being concerned with efficiency and/or equity. Therefore, you need to understand these crucial concepts and how they relate to health policy. So, before diving into the four principal questions, the first part of the book explores the concepts of efficiency and equity. First of all, though, a scene setting context of health care and health will be outlined.

Acknowledgements

First and foremost I want to acknowledge Paul Dolan for letting me draw heavily from our joint book *Distributing health care*, OUP, 2002. Without that book as a basis, I would not have started writing this one. Many thanks Paul, and thanks for supporting me to get on with it.

This book was written while spending a sabbatical year at The London School of Hygiene and Tropical Medicine. I am grateful to its Department of Public Health and Policy for providing me with work space, and to my colleagues there for many stimulating discussions.

I would like to thank Tony Culyer, Tor Iversen, Ivar Sønbø Kristiansen and Jon Magnussen for their comments on particular chapters, and Birgit Abelsen for providing Figures 1.3–6. The usual disclaimer applies.

Contents

Part 1 **The context of health and health care**

1 Health and health care *3*

   1.1 What is health? *3*

   1.2 What is health care? *6*

   1.3 What do health care and health do for people? *8*

   1.4 Health and health care across the world *11*

   1.5 Conclusion *14*

2 Economics and efficiency *17*

   2.1 More in means more out—but at a diminishing rate *19*

   2.2 Substitution: 'more than one way to skin a cat' *24*

   2.3 Scarcity: a dismal reality for the dismal science *32*

   2.4 Supply and demand—and the magic equilibrium *38*

   2.5 Conclusion *44*

3 What makes the market for health care different? *47*

   3.1 The perfect market model and the imperfect
       market for health care *47*

   3.2 Asymmetric information and the agency relationship *52*

   3.3 Externalities: selfishly motivated *55*

   3.4 Conclusion *59*

4 Equality and fairness *61*

   4.1 Externalities: *un*selfishly motivated *61*

   4.2 Transfers in cash or in kind *64*

   4.3 Three theories of distributive justice *67*

   4.4 The health frontier and trade-offs *72*

   4.5 Conclusion and some conceptual clarifications *77*

Part 2 **Intervening in the determinants of health**

5 The health environment *85*

   5.1 The physical environment *85*

   5.2 The social environment *89*

   5.3 Conclusion *92*

6 Health-related lifestyle *95*

    6.1 Diet *96*

    6.2 Exercise *98*

    6.3 Substance use *98*

    6.4 Conclusion *101*

Part 3 **Financing health care**

7 Uncertainty and health insurance *107*

    7.1 The welfare gain from insurance *108*

    7.2 Moral hazard *112*

    7.3 Risks differ: actuarially fair insurance *113*

    7.4 Adverse selection *114*

    7.5 Conclusion *116*

8 Compulsory insurance *119*

    8.1 Social health insurance *120*

    8.2 Tax-financed health care *121*

    8.3 Comparing three insurance systems *123*

    8.4 Conclusion *123*

9 Patient payment *127*

    9.1 The third party or the patient pays *128*

    9.2 Co-payment, co-insurance, co-funding, cost sharing *128*

    9.3 Deductibles *129*

    9.4 Distributive implications *131*

    9.5 Negative patient payments *132*

    9.6 Autonomous consumer or compliant patient *133*

    9.7 Conclusion *134*

Part 4 **Paying health care providers**

10 Primary care *139*

    10.1 Fee for service *140*

    10.2 Capitation *143*

    10.3 Salary *145*

    10.4 Comparing three payment systems *148*

    10.5 Conclusion *151*

11 Secondary care: reimbursing hospitals *153*

    11.1 Retrospective variable: cost reimbursement *154*

11.2 Prospective fixed budgets 155

11.3 Prospective variable 155

11.4 Macro vs micro level 157

11.5 Conclusion 157

12 Integrating the health care provider system 161

12.1 Combinations of payment systems in
primary and secondary care 161

12.2 The 'body' of the health care provider system 163

12.3 Interventions: integration and incentives 165

12.4 Conclusion 167

Part 5 **Economic evaluation and priority setting**

13 Non-monetary effects and monetary benefits 175

13.1 Incommensurable outcome measures 176

13.2 Commensurable measures of health effects 178

13.3 Production gains resulting from improved health 185

13.4 The monetary value of improved health 189

13.5 Threshold values and net monetary benefits 192

13.6 Conclusion 193

14 Costs and discounting 195

14.1 Average vs marginal costs 195

14.2 Identifying cost items: analysis viewpoint 199

14.3 Health service costs 200

14.4 Non-health service costs 200

14.5 The discount rate 201

14.6 Conclusion 205

15 Equity issues: going beyond CBA and ICER 207

15.1 Productivity changes and willingness to pay vary with income 207

15.2 Health gains: size and distribution matter 209

15.3 Severity: equality in prospective health 210

15.4 Age: equality in total health 210

15.5 Causes of ill health 213

15.6 Consequences beyond patients' health gains 214

15.7 Conclusion 215

References 219

Index 223

Part 1

The context of health and health care

Chapter 1

Health and health care

This first chapter considers what are meant by health and health care, as well as what health care does for people. The chapter is primarily an analytical one intended as scene setting for the later chapters. It includes some key figures to illustrate the wide differences in health, wealth, and health care spending across the world.

There is certainly more to life than health, in that people care about other things than their health alone. However, when in *ill* health, people care primarily about access to health care that can improve their health.

1.1 **What is health?**

Defining health is problematic and controversial. We can think of a continuum of definitions ranging from the very narrow to the very broad. At one extreme lies a narrow medico-technical definition, where health refers to the degree of bodily functioning that is observable to an external expert and measurable on medical instruments. At the other extreme lies the famous World Health Organization (WHO) definition of health as 'a state of complete physical, mental and social well-being, and not merely the absence of disease or infirmity'.

Such an all-encompassing definition of health would imply that everything becomes health care, simply because all commodities affect 'physical, mental and social well-being'. For the purposes of analysing principles of financing and distributing health care, a narrower concept of health is required. A pragmatic approach to finding a meaningful definition would be to look at how health is defined within the *generic descriptive systems* that are currently being used to measure health in clinical trials and evaluative studies. Interestingly, many of these descriptive systems refer to the concept of *health-related quality of life* (HRQL), implying something that is broader than the medico-technical definition of health but narrower than the WHO definition. But of course it still raises questions about what health means in the 'health-related' part of the phrase.

The different descriptive systems define health in different ways, largely because they are designed for different purposes. Condition-specific instruments are designed to measure health within a particular condition or disease group. Generic instruments have been developed to measure and compare health status across a range of different dimensions, although the dimensions often cannot be combined to form an overall single value for a composite health state. This is because the number of dimensions and/or levels within dimensions is very large. There now exist some descriptive systems that allow values to be attached to overall health status and, since these are suitable for use in informing resource allocation decisions across a range of diverse interventions, they will be the focus of attention here. Table 1.1 lists some of these

Table 1.1 Some generic descriptive systems that yield single index values for health

Descriptive system	Country of origin	Dimensions	Levels	Health states
EQ-5D (formerly EuroQol)	UK	Mobility, self-care, usual activities, pain/discomfort, anxiety/depression	3	243
Quality of well-being (QWB)	US	Mobility, physical activity, social functioning 27 symptoms/problems	3 2	1170
SF-6D (derived from SF-36)	UK (US)	Physical functioning, role limitations, social functioning, pain, mental health, vitality	4–6	18,000
Health utilities index: (HUI-III)	Canada	Vision, hearing, speech, ambulation, dexterity, emotion, cognition, pain	5–6	972,000
AQoL (Assessment of quality of life; or Australian QoL)	Australia	Illness, independent living, social relationships, physical senses, psychological well-being; each consists of three sub-dimensions	4	16.8 m
15D	Finland	Mobility, vision, hearing, breathing, sleeping, eating, speech, elimination, usual activities, mental function, discomfort/symptoms, depression, distress, vitality, sexual activity	5	30,518 m

descriptive systems together with the dimensions of health contained within them. The systems differ enormously in the dimensions that they include and also differ markedly in terms of where they are located on the 'narrow' to 'broad' spectrum. The HUI-III, for example, adopts a rather narrow 'within-the-skin' concept of health, whilst dimensions such as 'usual activities' puts the EQ-5D more towards the other end of the spectrum.

Even at this pragmatic level there are enormous differences in how health is defined. However, all the descriptive systems in Table 1.1 define it more narrowly than general well-being but much more widely than the presence or absence of a medical condition. Even so, they all seem to share a common understanding that health essentially deals with three key dimensions: *physical*, *mental*, and *social*, which corresponds with the WHO definition. The generic systems of Table 1.1 are more precise and descriptive about what these key dimensions would encompass.

The dimensions included in these descriptive systems refer to attributes of health *states* only. As such, they all refer to the 'quality' aspect of health as opposed to 'quantity', which takes account of the *duration*. Any meaningful metric of health would clearly have to include both quality and quantity.

A typical 'health span' can be illustrated in a quantity/quality space (Figure 1.1) as a stream of health, in which a particular HRQL is experienced in each time unit. When considered *ex ante*, it becomes probabilistic, with expected lifetime and expected health in each time unit. When each life year is weighted by the HRQL weight (usually ranging from 0 representing dead or worst imaginable health, to 1 representing best imaginable health), the area under the curve can be measured in terms of what WHO refers to as healthy life expectancy (HALE), defined as: 'average number of years that a person can expect to live in "full health" by taking into account years lived in less than full health due to disease and/or injury'.

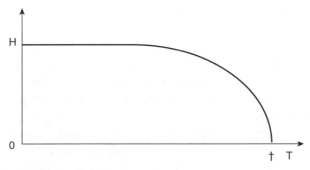

Fig. 1.1 The expected health span.

Imagine some given health capabilities, a given environment, and a completely health-neutral behaviour in which the individual does not engage in deliberately healthy or unhealthy activities; in these conditions the biological deterioration will follow a natural path.

Clearly, the shape of this 'health span' for the average person will vary across countries depending on the environment in which people live and their health-related lifestyle, as well as their health care use.

Thus, at the individual level, health gains are measured in terms of the expected increase in quality and quantity of life. These are normally expressed as quality-adjusted life years (QALYs) (see Chapter 13). At the population level, the more *people* that receive individual health gains, the higher the total health gains to society.

1.2 What is health care?

What make some types of resource use and some activities eligible to be termed 'health care' and others not? Health care refers to those resources society uses on people in ill health in an attempt to *cure* them or to *care* for them. In addition to curing and caring for people who have already become ill, health care includes some of those activities that seek to *prevent* people becoming ill in the first place. Beyond that, health care includes *rehabilitation* activities that are sometimes required after a more short-term intervention.

Cure is concerned with *improvements in health*. When a person's life is in danger, or when they suffer from an illness, a 'cure' might: i) fully restore that patient's health (e.g. rescue operations), ii) improve their health, though not completely (e.g. cataract operations), or iii) limit the extent to which health deteriorates (e.g. pain relief for the terminally ill). While the last situation might not correspond with the everyday connotation of the word 'cure', it is still motivated by improving health from what might otherwise be the case. Such situations might be referred to as palliative—or symptomatic—*treatments*. Palliation cloaks a disease.

Care is not directly concerned with improving health; rather it seeks *to provide dignity* for sick people. Certainly, there are important activities associated with providing care per se that are done to patients whilst at hospital receiving cure or treatments, but then care is already encompassed in what are referred to above as cure and treatment. When no known medical technologies are available that could cure or treat a person, caring is the only remaining activity that can be provided.

Prevention includes those resources whose main purpose is *to reduce the probability of illness or premature death*. In principle, prevention includes any intervention that seeks to reduce these risks; for example traffic, work, and environmental safety. As such, there are many ways in which illness and premature death can be prevented, many of which will lie outside our usual concepts of health care. The everyday connotation of prevention is that some undesired event can be *avoided*. However, at least in rich countries the vast majority of deaths represent the transition from chronic diseases: the final state can only be *postponed*. Hence, it might be more appropriate to consider many so-called 'prevention programmes' more as 'postponement programmes' that attempt to defer expected future adverse health events further into the future.

One pragmatic way to distinguish so-called 'preventive health care' from other preventive (or rather 'postponement') interventions is to say that for prevention to be termed health care, health professionals must be involved in its provision. An even more pragmatic approach would be to say that health care is whatever a national accounting system (e.g. the Organisation for Economic Co-operation and Development (OECD) system of classifying health care expenditures) defines it to be.

The types of health care identified above differ in at least three important respects. First, they differ in their *primary purpose*. Prevention, cure, and rehabilitation primarily seek to improve health; that is, *to produce health outcomes*. Caring, on the other hand, has a qualitatively different purpose. The interaction between a carer and a patient is not justified by its outcomes but by such process-related concepts as dignity, respect, autonomy, empathy, and sympathy. The economic evaluation of health care interventions has traditionally focused on the measurement of health outcomes and has largely ignored the less tangible, and consequently harder to measure, processes of care. Nonetheless, it is important to try to measure the 'goodness' from the various types of care since it is futile to take the view that all types of care are equally good.

Second, the types of health care differ according to the *availability of alternatives* to health care. There are clearly alternative measures to preventive health care. For example, in the case of anti-hypertensive drugs, there are alternative 'non-pharmacological' interventions such as reduced salt intake or physical exercise. If avoided deaths are 'produced' by prevention, then safety interventions might be better than health care at producing them. There are also substitutes for formal health care through the informal sector. Rather than being institutionalized, sick people could receive care from family members, friends, or charities. In the case of cure, however, there are very few—if any—substitutes. For most illnesses, most of us would prefer to see a health professional rather than anyone else. The extent to which alternatives to health care exist is crucial in the context of a discussion about the public provision of health care. In general, the fewer alternatives to health care that exist, the more vulnerable would people become simply because their own efforts will not help. Thus, we seem to feel a stronger duty for making health care freely available in such cases.

Finally, the types of health care differ according to their *time horizon*. Whilst both cure and care deal with the present, prevention is concerned with the future. The closer in time the relationship between the intervention and its consequent 'goodness', the more 'heroic' becomes the intervention, and the more morally obliged society becomes to make health care available. As a result, there is an ethical difference between health care that saves the life of a known individual (e.g. by mountain rescues) and health care that results in the saving of an unknown (statistical) life in the future (e.g. by road safety). Furthermore, there is an ethical difference between curing severely ill patients now and postponing expected future undesired events some time further into the future.

While cure may have a short time horizon in terms of hospital stay, for some diagnoses a long-term rehabilitation *after* the intervention would be crucial for its outcome. For example, after a cardiovascular event (such as a stroke) or an orthopaedic event (such as a kneecap fracture), intensive rehabilitation in terms of physiotherapy and patient efforts would be crucial. Unfortunately, a quick fix is not always an option!

1.3 **What do health care and health do for people?**

The reasons why people consume health care are very different from why they consume other goods and services. In general, consumers demand goods because of the pleasure (or avoided pain) these goods are expected to yield. In the language of economists and philosophers, consumers derive *utility* from the consumption of most goods and services. In more everyday language, we get satisfaction from consuming goods—otherwise we would not choose to spend money on them.

The reason why patients consume health care, however, is not because health care gives satisfaction per se, but rather because of the positive effect it has on health. Thus, the demand for health care is *derived* from the demand for health. However, the satisfaction per se that we may get from health care consumption is often negative. Health care might rather be considered a 'necessary evil' than what economists call a 'good'. The utilization of health care is associated with all sorts of disutility, from waiting time or the so-called side effects of medication through to the simple fact that most of us prefer to stay out of hospital. If it were not for the expected effects on health, we would prefer not to use health care. Hence, for people to be willing to consume health care, the benefits in terms of expected improvements in health must more than outweigh the disutility from the consumption of health care itself.

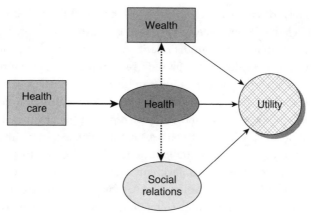

Fig. 1.2 The instrumental nature of health care and health.

So what good does good health do? First and foremost, good health has intrinsic value in its own right. There is a direct effect of improved health on the individual's utility or well-being. Beyond this direct effect, there are two important 'positive side effects' of improved health: healthy people are able to earn more, and are better able to satisfy their social needs. These relationships are shown in Figure 1.2. Health care and wealth are measurable in physical or monetary terms. Social relations can be measured in terms of number of friends and family members, as well as the frequency of contacts with them, but of course this says nothing about the quality of those contacts. Health can be measured by the various descriptive systems referred to above. Utility—measured in units of satisfaction, which economists refer to as 'utils'—is the hardest factor in Figure 1.2 to measure.

Consider first the right-hand side of Figure 1.2. Utility is what an individual would like to have the most of in life. To the left of utility are the three main classes of goods in life that yield utility: namely wealth, health, and social relations. Since more utility is preferred to less, more wealth, health, and social relations are also preferred to less. The popular saying, 'It's better to be rich and healthy than poor and sick' may suggest that only wealth and health matter, but human beings are social animals, and the more (and better) social relations we have, the better we feel. Of course, there may come a point when we have too much of a good thing—we become satiated—but most of us would prefer to be richer and healthier than poor and sick. And most of us would prefer to have a 'rich social life' including close friends, supportive family, and trusted colleagues and neighbours.

The arrows in Figure 1.2 illustrate the distinction between the *intrinsic* value of health (which bears directly on utility) and its *instrumental* value, i.e. via income and social life. Although we are not primarily concerned here with the functional relationship that each class of goods has on utility or well-being, nor with their relative importance, these issues appear to have some important health policy implications. On the relationship between wealth and utility, there is increasing evidence that above a certain income level more money does not make people happier. However, at low income levels, increased income certainly does make people happier. On the link between social relations and utility, what is important is that people feel that they *have* close friends, not how many friends they have. On the link between health and utility, such satiation is not suggested: more health is always better. Thus, the positive side effects of improved health on people's well-being are higher for poor people than for rich people, and higher for people who are socially isolated than for people who are not. This simple point shows the importance of going beyond the *measurement* of health when assessing the *importance* of health to people.

In general, we can make trade-offs between the classes of goods in life. For example, improved health can compensate for reduced wealth—it might be better to be poor and healthy than rich and sick. And pleasant social relations are a great compensation for reduced wealth—or would you rather be rich and lonely than poor but with many good friends?

Figure 1.2 shows the crucial roles that both health care and health play in life. As well as the direct arrow from health to utility, there are the dotted arrows from health to wealth, and from health to social relations. Of course, the interrelations between health, wealth, and social relations are more complex than the figure indicates. For example, it has been shown that good social relations have positive health effects, and that the social position associated with high income may also yield positive health effects. For simplicity, however, such effects are not included in this figure.

As noted above, when in need of cure, there are few—if any—substitutes to health care. Hence, access to health care is an important determinant of an individual's utility. Figure 1.2 also serves to highlight the important distinction between the sphere of interest of health professionals as compared to individual patients. The sphere of health professionals is—and should be—restricted to the arrow from health care to health. They are trained to have information on the expected health effects from various types of health care. Based on this information, then, it is the sphere of the patient to judge just how important a given health improvement is for their utility—provided, of course, that they have sufficient mental capabilities to do so.

Finally, consider the degree to which each of the factors in Figure 1.2 is measurable, as represented by the shape of the box for each factor. Utility, represented by the shaded circle, is certainly the hardest one to measure. At the other end of the spectrum are health care and wealth, which are more readily measurable in physical units or monetary terms. The ellipses for social relations and health occupy a middle ground.

1.4 **Health and health care across the world**

While general domestic product (GDP) is the most widely used indicator for 'the wealth of nations',[1] life expectancy (LE) at birth is the most commonly used indicator for 'the health of nations'. In general, the poorer a population is, the sicker it is and the shorter the average lifespan. However, the major causes of death are fundamentally different between rich and poor countries. In rich countries, the majority of people fulfil a complete lifespan (see Figure 1.1) and die from a chronic disease after the age of 70. In poor countries, death strikes at all ages following contagious diseases and malnutrition due to poverty.

The relationship between wealth and health suggests that poverty reduction has a significant impact on life expectancy, while, as Figure 1.3[2] shows, beyond a certain level further wealth increases have no further positive impact on longevity.

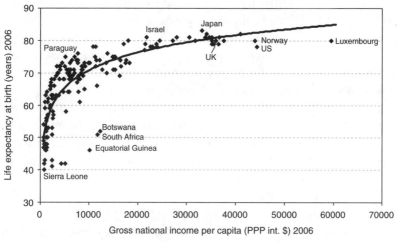

Fig. 1.3 The health by wealth relationship across the world.

---

[1] The phrase is also the abbreviated title of the best-known book in economics, by Adam Smith, published in 1776.

[2] Figures 1.3 to 1.6 are all based on a continuously updated data set provided by WHO (http://www.who.int/whosis/en/).

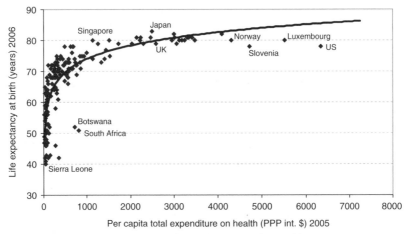

Fig. 1.4 The health by health care relationship across the world.

What about the effects of increased health care spending on improved health; does this show a more linear pattern? Figure 1.4 suggests much the same relationship as in Figure 1.3. At the bottom end, increased health care resources have tremendous impact on longevity. But once again, beyond a certain level there is hardly any positive link between increased health care spending and improved health. Of course, this should not be taken to imply that health care is ineffective at this level, but rather that health care is not the only determinant of longevity. While more health care would certainly improve the health of ill patients, there are other determinants of health that make people ill and hence in need of health care (see Part 2 of this book).

The curves in Figures 1.3 and 1.4 are so similar that they may suggest a linear relationship between a country's wealth and its health care spending. Is this the case; and does the relationship diminish or increase? Given the very strong impact of health care on health at the bottom end, poor countries would have better reason to spend relatively more of their GDP on health care than rich countries. As the major burdens of diseases due to poverty and malnutrition evaporate with increased wealth, one might think that increased health care spending is not as needed, which would suggest a *diminishing* proportion. However, Figure 1.5 gives a picture of *increasing* proportion of a country's wealth spent on health care.

The higher the GDP, the higher the proportion spent on health care. This phenomenon is observed not only in international comparisons across 168 countries, but also over time for most countries. In Norway, the proportion of GDP spent on health care has increased from 3% to 10% over the last 50 years.

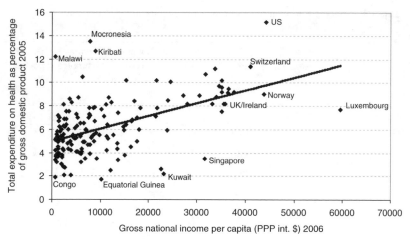

Fig. 1.5 The relationship between wealth and percentage of GDP spent on health care.

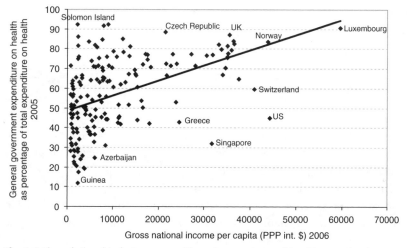

Fig. 1.6 The relationship between wealth and percentage of health care that is publicly financed.

It appears that the richer a country is, the more it can *afford* to spend on health care.

When countries become richer and can afford to spend relatively more on health care, does the pattern of how they finance their health care spending change? Yes, it does. Figure 1.6 shows that the richer a country gets, the more of its health care is tax financed. Interestingly, there are two separate characteristics when comparing countries with different levels of wealth. The richer the country, the smaller the proportion of health care financed directly from patients; and

Table 1.2 Differences in health, wealth and health care financing in some selected countries

	Life expectancy (years)	HC / capita $	HC /GDP %	Tax and social insurance %	Private insurance %	Out of pocket %
Countries						
US	78	6350	15	45	42	13
Norway	80	4307	9	84	1	15
UK	79	2597	8	87	1	12
Cuba	78	333	8	91	1	8
Haiti	61	71	6	51	5	44
Nigeria	48	45	4	4	9	87
India	63	100	5	19	5	76
Regions (average)						
Europe (n = 52)	75	1818	8	66	6	28
Africa (n = 46)	53	147	5	52	10	38
World average (n = 192)	67	810	6	59	8	33

Source: http://www.who.int/whosis/en/ Data from 2005 (2006 for life expectancies).

the more of the remainder that comes through some form of *public* rather than private insurance. In other words, the richer the country, the higher the proportion that is ex ante publicly financed.

Table 1.2 reveals sharp contrasts across some selected countries and regions. Life expectancies vary from around 80 years in rich countries to around 50 in Africa. In the 'world championship' in per capita health care spending, the USA is the big winner in that it spends close to 50% more than the second highest spender (Norway). When it comes to the distribution of funding, the USA is exceptional with its high share of private health insurance. Cuba is also exceptional: despite its low wealth, it has a high life expectancy and a high share of publicly funded health care. Its neighbour Haiti is the poorest country in the western hemisphere, with life expectancy and health care financing similar to Africa.

1.5 **Conclusion**

Rather than trying to find a definition of health in the theoretical literature, for the purpose of this book health is defined according to whatever descriptive system is chosen to look at the *changes* in health associated with different interventions. The primary concern in this book is with these *health gains* rather than with health per se.

Health care consists of four branches of activities: cure, care, prevention, and rehabilitation. Whilst health care personnel normally provide cure, care, and rehabilitation, prevention may involve a range of interventions whose overriding objective is to prevent ill health and reduce the risks of dying—of which only a part would be provided by the health sector. A pragmatic definition of health care, then, is whatever happens to be classified as such in a national accounting system. In this way, we avoid a controversial classification into what might clearly be termed health care and what might be referred to as cosmetics.

What can be done to improve health (i.e. reduce mortality and morbidity), and what can be done to reduce inequalities in health? You are not expected to be able to provide clear answers to these key public health issues. However, you may suspect that the answers have something to do with how health care resources are allocated in terms of efficiency and equity. Read on, and learn more about these concepts.

Suggested reading

WHO has plenty of relevant statistics: www.who.int/whosis/en/

OECD provides a great database on the economics of health for their 30 member countries: www.oecd.org

Williams, A. (1988) Priority setting in public and private health care: a guide through the ideological jungle. *Journal of Health Economics*, 7, 173–83.

Exercises

1. Which types of health care do you think have so little effect on people's health that they should not be termed *health* care?

2. Which types of ill health events can be *prevented*, and which can only be *postponed*?

3. Find the numbers for your country (or a country of your choice) in Table 1.2.

Chapter 2

Economics and efficiency

This chapter has the dual purpose of introducing the 'dismal science' of economics to non-economists, and of drawing trained economists' attention to those parts of their discipline that are most relevant in the context of this book.

Three main concepts are embodied in the heart of economics: production, distribution and scarcity. A short and precise definition can be found in *The Pocket Economist* (Pennant-Rea and Emmott, 1983): 'how scarce resources are used to produce and distribute goods and services to meet human wants'. Because one of its early practitioners, Thomas R. Malthus (1766–1834), believed that scarcity was so acute as to put the world permanently on the edge of famine, economics came to be known as the 'dismal science'.

Economists try to answer three questions simultaneously: what is to be produced, how is it to be produced, and for whom is it to be produced? As to the first question, most mainstream economists would say that people's preferences should determine what is to be produced, i.e. 'give the people what they want'. Alternatively, some would argue that people's needs should determine what is to be produced. This distinction between 'wants' (or 'desires') and 'needs' is particularly relevant in the context of health care, and is therefore something we shall return to. How things are to be produced depends on technology, as well as on the relative prices of the factors of production. Most economists would agree that a given level of a particular good or service should be produced in the cheapest way possible.

For whom they should be produced is an issue of distribution, and the answer given by conventional models is to distribute the goods according to people's willingness and ability to pay. This is how the problem of distribution is solved in model markets as well as in many real world markets. However, this distributive principle is more value laden than many economists would like to acknowledge. Interestingly, in those countries with publicly funded health care, an overriding objective is to distribute health care quite independently of people's willingness and ability to pay for such services.

When answering these fundamental questions, economic emerges as a field somewhere at the interface between engineering and ethics. Economists would ask engineers about what is technologically feasible, i.e. how can we possibly produce the things that people want or need? And they would ask politicians about which distributive principle society would like as a basis for determining who is to have these things. Thus, when the technologies have been identified and the distributive principles have been decided, the economist springs into action.

Economic models have three types of building blocks: i) identities, ii) technological relations, and iii) the objective function. A typical identity relationship is the account balance: 'money out = money in'. In other words, the revenues obtained from selling the good are equal to the costs of purchasing the input factors plus any profits.

A technological relationship would be a production function that explains the relationship between input factors and output.

Since an optimal allocation of resources crucially depends on what we want to achieve, all economic models must also have an objective function, even if this is only stated implicitly. This objective function must also specify the appropriate distribution of resources in question. For instance, if we want to maximize health, then health care would be allocated differently from how it would be allocated if the objective were to do the most good for the most severely ill.

In dealing with each of these building blocks, economic models make a number of assumptions about the way in which inputs and outputs relate to one another and how producers and consumers behave. Producers are assumed to maximize profit; in order to do so, they must organize their production in the most cost-effective way. In competitive markets, this behaviour is forced upon producers because they could go out of business if they did not maximize profits. However, in non-competitive markets, producers are not similarly forced.

Identity and technological relationships are considered to be positive issues whilst stating the objective function, and the distributive principles are normative issues. Positive issues deal with how things are, while normative issues deal with how things ought to be. This distinction between positive and normative is very important and is often strongly emphasized in economics.

However, economists may have different views as to which parts of their models they should label positive and which normative.

In the particular context of applying economic models to inform health policy, it is for society to state the objectives and the principles under which health care should be distributed. These are therefore clearly normative issues, which might narrow the degrees of freedom that economists have when choosing which types of models to use. Beyond these explicit policy issues, there are often implicit normative issues hidden in the economic models we use. An admittedly normative statement here is to say that analysts should be honest and explain any such distributive implications of their models.

Our discipline is usually divided between 'macroeconomics' and 'microeconomics', as can be seen from the titles of most introductory textbooks in economics. Although the boundaries between macro- and microeconomics are often quite blurred, the majority of health economics appears to have its theoretical basis in microeconomics. Microeconomics focus on the behaviour of market actors, and analyse how their behaviour influences supply and demand and hence prices and quantities.

Starting from basics, the actors in the market are usually referred to as 'producers' and 'consumers', sometimes as firms and households, or simply as sellers and buyers. Producers are assumed to be 'only in it for the money', i.e. they are motivated by maximizing profits. Their behaviour is constrained by technology as well as by prevailing market prices. Under 'perfect competition' each producer is a 'price taker'; that is, their quantities are so small relative to the size of the market that they do not individually influence market prices. However, under other market forms, a single producer may influence the market price, as would be the case under monopoly. Consumers are assumed to be 'only in it for the pleasure', i.e. they are motivated by maximizing utility. Their choices are constrained by their income and the prevailing market prices. The moves they make depend on their individual 'taste'; some like it hot, some like it mild. The following sections explain some important aspects of microeconomic models.

2.1 More in means more out—but at a diminishing rate

2.1.1 Production functions

A production function sets out the technology relationship, explaining how the amounts of input factors, such as labour and machinery, vary with the production of goods. Usually we find that production increases with more inputs, although it rarely increases proportionally with input. Initially, production would often increase more than the increase in input, and we have what are termed 'economies of scale'. After some level of production, this 'over-proportional' increase starts to diminish to the point where there is 'constant return to scale', i.e. production increases proportionally with input. After this level, there is 'under-proportional' increase: production increases at a diminishing rate. The good thing, though, is that production still increases with more input. But most good things come to an end, i.e. there comes a point where more input does not yield more output (termed the 'satiation point'), after which more input would actually reduce the level of output. Figure 2.1 illustrates this pattern, where the horizontal axis, labelled *L*, is the amount of labour used, and the vertical axis, *X*, is the amount of goods produced.

The S-shaped production function has been identified across very different types of production: different goods and services, different input factors, as well as different technological developments. It is no surprise, therefore, that it has intuitive appeal. Consider doctors as an input factor in a hospital equipped with various types of machinery. One doctor would spend much time running from one end of the building to the other. Employing more doctors would mean that less time would be wasted. And, when doctors specialize their skills across diagnosis and patient groups (e.g. oncology, paediatrics), this specialization and task division will increase production at a higher rate than the increase in number of doctors.

However, when wasted time has been saved and there is no more room for specialization, more doctors may still lead to increased production, but at a

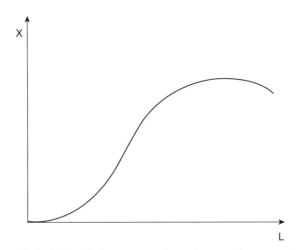

Fig. 2.1 The typical relationship between one input factor and output.

diminishing rate. There then comes a point beyond which more doctors would get in each other's way, so that production would actually fall.

The central concept of productivity must not be forgotten here. This can be defined on an average or marginal basis. Average productivity is simply the total output divided by the number of units of the particular input: in the case of labour, it means X / L. Marginal productivity is the additional output which follows from employing an additional unit of the particular input: in the case of labour, it means $\Delta X / \Delta L$ where Δ (delta, from the Greek alphabet) means change. The average or marginal productivity depends crucially on the extent to which other inputs are involved. Labour productivities would normally be higher the more machinery there is behind each employee. So, as well as different paces of work, differences in labour productivity across countries may also be due to differences in how much machinery is available.

As to the optimal number of workers to employ, not much can be said on the basis of this general production function alone. The only thing we can say for sure is not to employ beyond the satiation point at which new workers would only mess things up. The number of workers to employ will depend on the price of the input (the wage) and the price of the goods (as well as on the level and relative price of capital). The good thing about such production functions is that the relationships they are based upon can actually be measured in physical units. As such, they differ from utility functions, to which we now turn.

Productivity in a hospital ward

A hospital ward has many input factors. Imagine a ward where only *one* input factor (employees) varies with activity. In Table 2.1, L refers to the number of doctors on each shift and X is the number of patients operated on. The third column, X / L, expresses *average productivity*, which happens to increase up to the fourth doctor employed, and diminishes after the fifth. The final column expresses *marginal productivity* ($\Delta X / \Delta L$), i.e. how much the production changes as a result of increasing the use of input by one unit. In this example, the first doctor increases the production by 4; the second doctor increases the production by 6 (from 4 to 10); and employing a third doctor leads to an increased total production of 10—which is where the marginal productivity is highest. Up until the seventh doctor, the marginal productivity is positive, though diminishing. If the eight doctor is employed, then total production falls, i.e. this doctor has a *negative* marginal productivity.

Productivity in a hospital ward *(continued)*

Table 2.1 Input, output, *average* productivity and *marginal* productivity

L	X	X /L	ΔX / ΔL
0	0	0	
			4
1	4	4	
			6
2	10	5	
			10
3	20	6, 7	
			8
4	28	7	
			7
5	35	7	
			5
6	40	6, 7	
			2
7	42	6	
			–2
8	40	5	

Exercise

Use the numbers in the first two columns to draw a curve (like Figure 2.1) that illustrates how much production we get from increased labour.

Find the points on the curve where the *average* productivity is highest and where the *marginal* productivity is highest.

2.1.2 **Utility functions**

A utility function sets out the relationship between the amounts of various goods consumed and the utility that a consumer derives from them. The general relationship between the units of a particular good consumed and utility (holding other goods constant) is assumed to be somewhat simpler than with the production function above. Utility increases with more units consumed, but again at a diminishing rate. After a satiation point, the utility begins to fall. See Figure 2.2, where the horizontal axis, labelled X, is the amount of a good consumed, and the vertical axis, U, is the utility that the consumer derives.

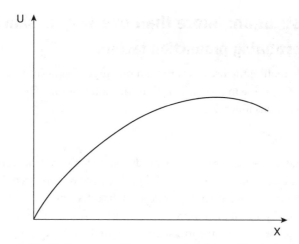

Fig. 2.2 The relationship between units consumed and the utility derived.

Most people will agree with the general shape of this utility function. For any good you consume (e.g. chocolate), the amount of satisfaction you get from succeeding units of that good diminishes. This is sometimes referred to as 'the law of diminishing marginal utility'. And after a certain level (again referred to as the satiation point), you realise that you wish you had not had the last unit. The average utility is simply the total amount of utility enjoyed divided by the number of units consumed to get that amount of utility: U/X. Marginal utility is then defined as the additional utility one gets from an extra unit of the particular good: $\Delta U/\Delta X$. And it is the concept of marginal utility that is most useful, because it is the pleasure you expect to get from an extra unit that determines how much you are willing to give up (most often in terms of money) in order to get it.

Unfortunately, it is hard to measure utility in any meaningful unit. Whilst you might be able to attach relative utilities to additional units of a good (e.g. 'the second chocolate gave half the satisfaction of the first one'), it is difficult, if not impossible, to express absolute levels of utility. The way in which a consumer's utility is usually measured is through their willingness to pay for the particular unit. Holding everything else constant, the more a consumer is willing to pay for a good, the more utility they are considered to get from that good.

But, of course, an individual's willingness to pay will be related to their income. A rich person might be willing to spend more on a chocolate than a poor person, not necessarily because the rich person gets greater utility from the chocolate but simply because they can afford to pay more for it. So the way conventional economic theory measures how much utility a consumer gets is by an income-dependent metric, i.e. money.

2.2 **Substitution: 'more than one way to skin a cat'**

2.2.1 **Substituting production factors**

Most goods require the use of more than one input factor in the production process. In the following, we will stick to the conventional factors of labour and capital (or machinery):

$$X = f(L, K) \qquad (2.1)$$

Suppose that a given quantity, X_0, is produced with a particular combination of labour and capital, L_0 and K_0, and that the marginal productivity of each factor is positive (i.e. we are not at or beyond the satiation point). If we were to reduce labour by a certain amount ($L_1 < L_0$) while still maintaining the initial quantity, X_0, we would have to use more capital ($K_1 > K_0$). Equally, if less capital were to be used ($K_2 < K_0$), we would have to employ more labour ($L_2 > L_0$) in order to maintain X_0.

Thus, by identifying all combinations of labour and capital which produce a given quantity, an isoquant (= equal quantity) can be depicted. In Figure 2.3, the horizontal axis indicates the amount of labour, L, and the vertical axis the amount of capital, K. The three combinations of labour and capital are shown as points on the isoquant that produce output X_0.

The downward slope of the isoquant shows that, if we use less of one input factor, we would have to compensate for this by using more of the other factor. The isoquant is convex because of diminishing marginal productivity. When we use a lot of one factor, the succeeding units of it are less productive

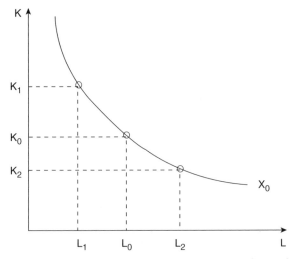

Fig. 2.3 A given quantity produced with various combinations of input factors.

than the preceding units. Hence, we would have to use an increasing number of extra units in order to compensate for a reduced unit of the alternative factor. At the same time as the alternative factor is being reduced, we forgo a higher and higher marginal productivity the more we reduce it.

So why was it necessary to trouble you with isoquants? First, because it is important to remember that there is more than one way to skin a cat, more than one way to save a life, and certainly more than one way to treat an illness. Admittedly, the number of alternative options are not so many that they can be identified on a continuous smooth and elegant isoquant, but in most instances it is feasible to choose between alternative technologies, or different combinations of inputs, in health care.

Second, isoquants help to explain two levels of efficiency. There is technical efficiency, which means that a combination on the isoquant is chosen. This means that we do not waste input factors. All points on the isoquant represent technically efficient combinations. If a point to the north-east of the isoquant were chosen to produce the same quantity, we would be using more input factors than necessary. It would then be possible to reduce the amount of labour and/or capital without reducing the quantity produced.

Which point on the isoquant should you choose? The answer is to choose the cheapest combination of inputs, which refers to the second level of efficiency: cost efficiency. The exact point chosen on the isoquant will depend on the relative prices of the input factors. In Figure 2.4, a budget line (or 'isocost' = equal costs) has been added to illustrate the relative prices of labour and capital.

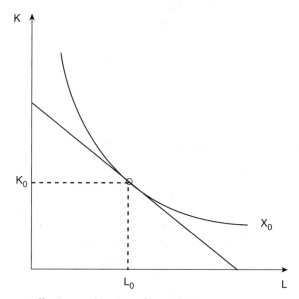

Fig. 2.4 The cost-effective combination of input factors.

The cost-efficient point is where the budget line is tangential to the isoquant. At that point only would the given quantity be produced most cheaply. Any other point on the isoquant represents a combination of input factors that involve higher total costs.

If wages increase, the budget line becomes steeper and labour would be substituted with capital. Conversely, if capital costs were to increase, the line becomes flatter and capital would be substituted with labour. The budget line in Figure 2.4 is tangential to the point (L_0, K_0), showing this to be the most cost-efficient combination of labour and capital.

Of course, much depends on the time period over which decisions are made. In the short run, with buildings and machinery installed, it may be hard to suddenly opt for an alternative technology. Consequently, most economics textbooks assume that in the short run, capital is a fixed factor of production whilst labour is a variable factor. In the long run, there is more discretion about which point on the isoquant to choose since both capital and labour are assumed to be variable. Precisely when the short run finishes and the long run starts is rarely defined; they are simply conceptual devices.

When comparing the choice of technology between countries, we find that where labour is cheap, more of it is used relative to capital. In rich countries, on the other hand, where labour is expensive, firms tend to use relatively more capital in the production process. This is true of health care as well.

The discussion above had the starting point: a given quantity, X_0 (depicted as a point on the isoquant), is to be produced; how can we do this most cheaply? An alternative starting point is: we have a given budget; how can we produce as much as possible? The answers to both questions take us to points that are cost efficient.

An important reminder: the expression 'maximum quantity for the minimum cost' simply does not make sense. (If you write that in the exam, you would fail!) Either we maximize production for a given budget or we minimize costs for a given quantity of production.

2.2.2 Substituting consumption goods

Even the saddest child can be compensated when he has to give up a toy. Give him a different toy or an ice cream, and you observe the simple point: if you have to forgo a unit of one good, the lost utility (or well-being, satisfaction, or happiness) can be compensated by the utility obtained from more of the other good that is made available. Analogous to the fact that there is more than one way to skin a cat, there is certainly more than one way to get some satisfaction.

Alternative input combinations

The first column of the table below indicates that the production level is the same ($X = 10$) no matter which of the listed combination of input factors is chosen. The next two columns show the technically efficient alternative combinations of labour, L, and capital, K.

Exercise 1

Put the numbers in these columns into a figure of the type illustrated in Figure 2.3.

The final column shows the costs of the alternative combinations, when one employee costs $200 and one machine $400 per day. Hence, it shows the required budget for choosing the various combinations.

Table 2.2 Alternative input combinations with their associated total costs

X	L	K	Costs in $ (200 L + 400 K)
10	1	6	2,600
10	2	4	2,000
10	3	3	1,800
10	4	2, 4	1,760
10	5	2	1,800
10	6	1, 75	1,900

Exercise 2

Identify the cost-effective combination, and draw a budget line that is tangential to this point, where the slope shows the relative prices of labour and capital.

Alternative input combinations, II

Table 2.3 shows technically efficient combinations for production $X = 15$, as well as their costs.

Exercise

Draw this new isoquant into the same figure as in the exercise above, and draw the budget line that is tangential to the cost-effective combination.

Table 2.3 Alternative input combinations with their associated total costs II

X	L	K	Costs in $ (200 L + 400 K)
15	1	12	5,000
15	2	8	3,600
15	3	6	3,000
15	4	4, 7	2,680
15	5	4	2,600
15	6	3, 7	2,680

Imagine a hospital ward with a given budget of $2,600, which currently is spent on the input combination $1L$ and $6K$. Table 2.2 shows that this gives a production $X = 10$. However, note that this point lies on the budget line you have just drawn: a line that is tangential to the isoquant $X = 15$. Thus, it would then be possible to increase the production from 10 to 15 by getting rid of 2 machines, and use the cost savings ($800) on 4 additional employees.

Inputs and outputs in the context of health care and health

How *measurable* are the parameters included in the following general production function?

$$X = f \text{(labour, capital, raw material, etc)} \tag{2.2}$$

Clearly, input factors are measurable in terms of man hours (labour), machinery and buildings (capital), water (raw material), etc. Output, however, may not always be that easy to measure. While physical goods (e.g. building bricks) can easily be measured, some softer types of services might be more difficult, in that they are not always homogeneous (e.g. haircuts can be counted, but they differ). When it comes to health care, and health, things are getting even more difficult—as you might expect.

First, there is the production function with health care as the output, simply replacing X with *HC*. For a certain type of health care, i, the production function, may be expressed as:

$$HC_i = f_i (\text{doctors, nurses, drugs, etc}) \tag{2.3}$$

While the *quality* of *HC* certainly differs, the *quantity* is increasingly being measured, e.g. in terms of resource-adjusted hospital admissions (more in Chapter 11).

Second, there is a 'production function' at a subsequent, and qualitatively different, level, that of using health care to 'produce' health:

$$H = f(HC) \tag{2.4}$$

While you may dislike the connotation of 'producing' health, the important point to accept here is that health care resources are being used to have a positive effect on people's health, and therefore it is crucial to measure how much health improvement can be achieved in different patient groups by the use of different medical technologies (more in Chapter 13).

Consider a simplified and typical utility function, where a consumer gains utility, U, from the two goods, X and Y:

$$U = u(X, Y) \tag{2.5}$$

Imagine that a particular combination of the two goods X_0 and Y_0 yields a given level of satisfaction, U_0. If the individual has to give up one unit of X, some more of Y is required in compensation. The minimum compensation required in order to remain at the initial utility level is that which brings him to Y_1:

$$U_0 = u(X_0, Y_0) = u(X_1, Y_1) \tag{2.6}$$

Figure 2.5 illustrates an indifference curve that shows those combinations of two goods that yield a given level of utility for a particular consumer. (Note the similarities with isoquants that show those combinations of two inputs that yield a given output.)

Indifference curves slope downwards from left to right: in order to remain equally happy, less Y requires more X. And like isoquants, indifference curves are convex to the origin. The reason lies in the concept mentioned above, that

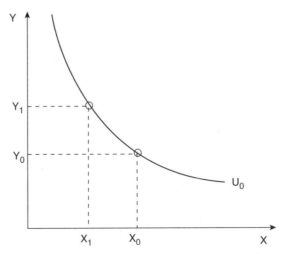

Fig. 2.5 A given utility level obtained from various combinations of two goods.

of diminishing marginal utility. The more you get of one good, the less additional utility you get from each extra unit, and so you require more of it to compensate you for the loss of the other good. At the same time, the less you get of the other good, the higher is the lost utility from each additional unit forgone, and so you require even more of the other good in compensation. The slope of the curve illustrates the consumer's marginal rate of substitution between X and Y, (MRS_{XY}), i.e. the number of Y required for being willing to forgo one additional X.

What is so special about indifference curves apart from their elegance? The answer is that they illustrate probably the most important attribute of consumer behaviour, namely that we make trade-offs. Such trade-offs are made between apples and oranges, between fruit and chocolate, between food and wine, between cars and holidays, and, not least, between wealth and health.

Unfortunately, indifference curves are not observable and cannot be measured in the same way as isoquants. Rather, indifference curves are mental constructions—at least within the minds of economists. They crucially reflect the taste of the given consumer. Human beings are uniquely different, and consumers are sovereign in expressing their tastes. Thus, while some consumers may appear to have pretty weird preference structures, there is no 'right' or 'wrong' shape to their indifference curves.

However, there are some restrictions that economists impose on just how weird an individual's preference function can be. One of the most important restrictions is that preferences must be transitive. This means that if you prefer A to B and B to C, then you should also prefer A to C. So, if we know you

'It's better to be rich and healthy than poor and sick.'

Of course we all agree with this popular saying, simply because it is a choice that doesn't involve trade-offs. Good health is always preferred to less good health, and more income is usually preferred to less income. But is it better to be rich and sick than poor and healthy? Well, that all depends on *how* sick and *how* poor you are, and your preferences between the two. Some people have expensive tastes, while some are health freaks, so the trade-off between the two goods would differ. Anyway, the conception of this trade-off between wealth and health can be illustrated by an indifference curve in the 'wealth—health space' of Figure 2.6.

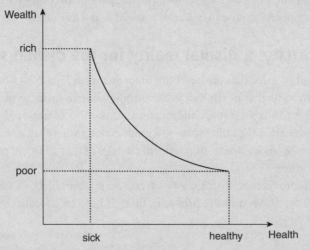

Fig. 2.6 Trade-offs in the wealth—health space.

The *slope* of the curve at any given point would then be the marginal rate of substitution of wealth for health *(MRS$_{WH}$)*, or how much *W* you are pre-pared to forgo in order to get one additional unit of *H* at a particular point on the curve. The *shape* of the curve reflects the same general preference structure as in Figure 2.5 above: the less you have of a particular good, in this case *H*, the more you would be willing to give up of the other good, in this case *W*, in order to get an extra unit of *H*. Hence, the more sick you are, the more money you would be willing to sacrifice in order to gain a given level of health improvement.

prefer hot dogs to hamburgers and hamburgers to pizza, then we can infer that you prefer hot dogs to pizza. If you did not, then you would be an irrational consumer.

Given all these combinations of goods that yield the same level of utility, which one would the consumer choose? The answer, analogous to that for production, is that they would choose the cheapest combination, which will be determined by the relative prices of the goods in question. In Figure 2.7, the budget line illustrates the relative prices of X and Y. The budget line is tangential to the indifference curve at (X_0, Y_0) and here the consumer maximizes utility.

If the price of X increases (or the price of Y falls), the budget line becomes steeper and the consumer would substitute X with more of Y. If the price of X falls (or the price of Y increases), the budget line becomes flatter and the consumer would choose to consume more of X and less of Y.

2.3 **Scarcity: a dismal reality for the dismal science**

Had it not been for the constraints on input factors in Figure 2.4, society could have moved further north-east in the output space in order to increase production. And were it not for budget constraints, most of us would fly off further north-east in the utility space to a utopian point where satiation is reached for all the goods we desire. But, unfortunately, we face scarcity of resources in the real world.

Most input factors, such as raw materials, capital, and labour, have limited availability. The economic problem, then, is how to allocate the available

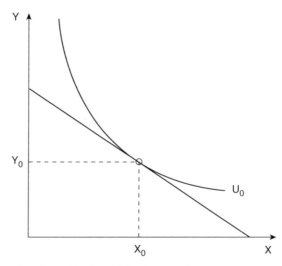

Fig. 2.7 The preferred combination of the two goods.

inputs across different sectors or firms that produce different goods. Consider the typical model of two input factors: labour and capital, which are available in fixed quantities, L_0 and K_0. These input factors can be used for producing either of two goods: X and Y.

If all inputs were used to produce X, there would be nothing left to produce Y, and vice versa. Imagine that we start by producing only Y. If one less unit of Y is produced, the factors required to produce this unit would be released and could be reallocated to produce as many units of X as possible. The production of Y could be reduced still further, thus transferring more and more factors to the production of X. What emerges, then, is another elegant curve: the production possibility frontier (PPF), or transformation curve, as shown in Figure 2.8.

The reason for its downward slope is that more input factors devoted to the production of Y mean fewer input factors devoted to the production of X; more units of Y produced mean fewer units of X produced. The PPF is concave to the origin because of diminishing marginal productivities for each of the factors of production. Incremental units of labour and capital devoted to the production of Y will produce fewer additional units of Y. As inputs are taken away from the production of X, more and more units of X will have to be forgone in order to produce fewer and fewer additional units of Y.

The terms PPF and transformation curve are indicative of what the curve in Figure 2.8 shows. They also capture concepts that lie at the heart of economics. The PPF indicates the maximum amount of one good that can be produced given the amount of the other good that is produced. The collection of frontier

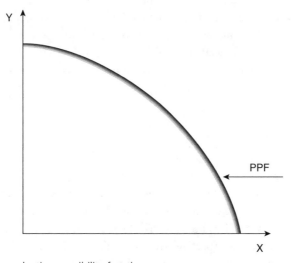

Fig. 2.8 The production possibility frontier.

points is referred to as being Pareto-efficient. This means that, at any point on the frontier, it is not possible to increase the production of one good without also reducing the production of the other good. Clearly, points inside the frontier cannot be Pareto-efficient. If we are inside the PPF, it would be possible to move to a point on the frontier by increasing the production of one good without reducing the production of the other.

The alternative name for the PPF—the transformation curve—literally suggests that (the production of) one good can be transformed into (the production of) the other good. This is achieved by withdrawing input factors from the production of one good and putting them into the production of the other good. Hence, the alternative to producing an extra unit of one good is what might otherwise have been produced of the other good. The slope of the transformation curve illustrates the marginal rate of transformation between X and Y (MRT_{XY}). What we forgo in terms of lost production of the other good is referred to as the *opportunity cost* of producing an extra unit of one good. The shape of the curve in Figure 2.8 tells us that the opportunity cost of producing incremental units of X increases, i.e. more and more units of Y have to be forgone for each additional unit of X that is produced.

A frontier point is always superior to an interior point, but which frontier point should we choose? That all depends on the preferences of the consumer: if they have a strong preference for X over Y, then more of X should be produced, and vice versa. The point at which an individual consumer's indifference curve is tangential to the PPF is exactly where their utility is maximized, as shown in Figure 2.9.

At point E, the given amounts of the factors of production have been allocated between the production of the two goods so as to reflect what people want. This unique combination of the two goods corresponds with allocative efficiency. This top-level efficiency requires that the marginal rate of transformation between X and Y (MRT_{XY}) is equal to the consumer's marginal rate of substitution between X and Y (MRS_{XY}). If unequal, it is possible to bring about a Pareto improvement. For example, if $MRT_{XY} = 2$ and $MRS_{XY} = 1$, then the economy can transform one X into two Y. Since individuals are indifferent between one X and one Y, by producing two more units of Y and one less unit of X, one individual can be made better off.

Many microeconomics textbooks include models in which two consumers trade with two different sets of goods, whose total quantities are given and whose distribution between the two consumers has been randomly determined 'like manna from heaven'. It is unlikely that the individuals' initial bundles would correspond with their respective tastes for the goods. However, by voluntarily exchanging goods with each other, an optimal distribution can be achieved.

The opportunity cost of health care

In almost any discussion with health economists you can expect to hear them using the concept of opportunity cost, so you might as well be introduced to some of the contexts in which the concept is used. Opportunity cost essentially refers to the *benefits forgone* in the best alternative programme to which the resources might otherwise have been allocated. There are some interesting connotations to consider. When you hear the word 'cost', there is a negative connotation, in that it reminds us that nothing comes for free, and we need to find out if we can afford it. In contrast, 'benefit' has a positive connotation—in that all resource use can potentially create benefit in terms of more utility, well-being, or health. Therefore, 'always look on the bright side of life' by remembering: opportunity costs = benefits forgone!

At the most aggregate national level, there are always other goods and services on which resources can be allocated. If a society would prefer to spend 15% rather than 10% of GDP on health care, the opportunity cost of that extra spending is the benefits forgone, e.g. less private consumption goods.

At the public sector level, the ministry of finance is always faced with competing alternatives to health care, e.g. education. The cost of an additional billion on health care can be measured in terms of the forgone benefits that this sum of money would have created in terms of more teachers or better teaching facilities.

At the health sector level, the alternative to spending an extra million on a hospital would be the health benefits that the same sum of money would yield in primary care.

At the hospital level, managers would be familiar with fights over budgets, listening to arguments from competing wards about the potential benefits for *their* patients of an additional slice of the hospital budget.

At the GP level, the doctor knows perfectly well that the extra time spent on the patient in front of them involves less time for the patient in the waiting room. So what are the benefits forgone to the one waiting outside?

Hence, the underlying ethics in the concept of opportunity cost resembles realities we simply cannot escape from: resources spent on the programme under consideration would always have alternative uses. Are the benefits from this programme better than the best alternative? If yes, then implement the programme. If no, then go for the best alternative. It is as simple as that.

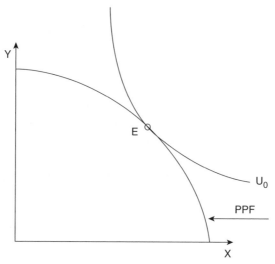

Fig. 2.9 The PPF and utility maximization.

Since the exchange is voluntary, neither of them would be made worse off than when they started, but their relative utility gains would depend on their relative negotiation skills. With a sufficient number of exchanges between the two individuals, a curve of optimal distribution will result.

Based on this curve, a frontier can be derived that depicts the optimal distribution of the goods between the two individuals: the utility possibility frontier (UPF) in Figure 2.10. The UPF shows all points where Pareto optimality exists, i.e. at any point on the frontier it is not possible for one individual to increase their utility without the other individual having to reduce theirs. Clearly, points inside the frontier cannot be Pareto-optimal. The shape of the UPF will be determined by the extent to which the two individuals are able to generate utility from the goods they consume. The precise point on the UPF that is reached will depend on the initial distribution of goods between the two individuals and on their relative bargaining skills.

The frontier intersects the axes in two extreme distribution points. At U_A^{max}, A's utility is maximized by consuming everything available of the two goods (nothing left for B). The other extreme is at U_B^{max}, where B has got it all. At least two important things should be said about the UPF. First, it is based on individualistic utility functions, which means that each individual is concerned only with their own utility, something that is obtained from their own consumption of goods. Second, the UPF in itself offers no guidelines as to the ranking of preferred distributions. All points are equally 'optimal' according to the Pareto criterion, even the most extreme points.

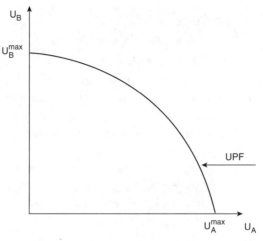

Fig. 2.10 The utility possibility frontier.

The health possibility frontier HPF

Analogous to the *production* possibility frontier (PPF) and the *utility* possibility frontier (UPF), we shall introduce the concept of a *health* possibility frontier (HPF). Rather than utility, health is on the two axes. And, rather than thinking about a given total basket of goods that are to be shared between two consumers, we now think of a given total health care budget (or a given set of health care resources, e.g. doctor hours) shared between

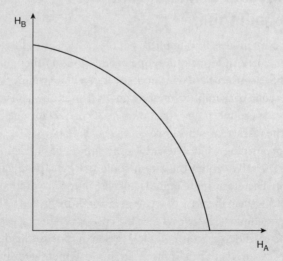

Fig. 2.11 The health possibility frontier.

The health possibility frontier HPF—*(continued)*

two patients. If all health care were allocated to patient A, it would yield (or 'produce') $H_A{}^{max}$ for A, and no health gains for B. At the other extreme, if all health care were given to B, they would gain it all at $H_B{}^{max}$.

The health frontier is, in principle, easier to measure than the utility frontier. The shape of the curve reflects diminishing marginal productivity of health care on health, i.e. the more health care that is allocated to A, the less additional health is produced. Note that the more of the total health care resources we have allocated to A, the higher is the opportunity cost in terms of forgone health improvements to B.

This HPF is a very helpful analytical device and extremely important—in that it highlights that the opportunity costs of improving one person's health can be measured by the sacrifice in terms of other patients' forgone health. This frontier visualises scarcity applied to health care. Note also that all points on the frontier are Pareto-efficient, in that it is impossible to improve one person's health without reducing that of another person.

Given that the health frontier has identified all efficient combinations of health for the two persons, the question is: *which* point on the curve is the preferred one? That all depends on one's views on equity and fairness, something to be discussed in Chapter 4.

2.4 Supply and demand—and the magic equilibrium

From the above models, it is implied that the more we produce of one good, the more it 'costs' in terms of forgone production of other goods. And the more you have consumed of one good, the less you are willing to pay for it in terms of forgone consumption of other goods. Let us now consider the interaction between producers and consumers in the market for one good in isolation from the market for other goods.

When considering what determines the supply of good X, we begin by reminding ourselves about the diminishing marginal productivity of each input factor. Therefore, more input factors are needed to produce each incremental unit X. When the price of an input factor is unaffected by how much of it a producer employs, it follows that the cost of producing each additional unit will increase. Beyond this 'technical reason' for increasing marginal costs, there might be an 'input price reason' in that an input factor might become more expensive the more of it that is employed. In general, then, it seems reasonable to assume that producers are faced with increasing marginal costs.

Because each producer is assumed to try to maximize profits, they will not sell any unit of output at a loss, at least not in the long run (in the short run, they might be able to sustain losses providing these are covered by increased subsequent profits). If the market price is higher than the cost of producing the last unit, the producer will expand production; hence supply increases. Conversely, if the market price is lower than the marginal costs of production, supply will be reduced. As a result, the long-run supply curve is identical to the marginal cost curve. By aggregating each producer's supply curve, we have the market supply curve. The higher the market price, the higher the market supply.

We noted earlier that a consumer is prevented from reaching their satiation point by their income and the price of the good. If a consumer is willing (and able) to pay more for an additional unit of the good than its prevailing market price, then they will buy it. If their willingness to pay for the good is less than the market price, they will not buy it. The maximum amount a consumer is willing to pay for an extra unit of the good signals how much they value the benefits from that extra unit.

In general, each consumer is assumed to have a demand curve that reflects how much they value incremental units of the good. The amount that each of us demands at a given price will depend on our income and on our preferences. But it seems reasonable to assume that if the price of a good were to fall, we would be more inclined to buy an extra unit of the good. Analogous to the above aggregation to determine a market supply curve, when we aggregate each consumer's demand curve, we have the market demand curve. The lower the market price, the higher the market demand.

Figure 2.12 illustrates the typical market with an upward-sloping supply curve, S, and a downward-sloping demand curve, D. The horizontal axis is the quantity of the good, X, and the vertical axis is the price, P. The intersection between S and D determines the equilibrium price, p^*, and quantity, X^*. At this point, the cost to producers of the last unit is exactly equal to the value that consumers place on this unit. For many economists, this represents Nirvana!

The curves in Figure 2.12 could be relatively steep or relatively flat. There are several factors that influence the steepness of the supply curve. These include: i) the time period: in the short run, supply curves are relatively steep due to the existence of fixed factors that limit the scope for increased output, whilst in the long run, supply curves are flatter because all factors are assumed to be variable; ii) factor mobility: the greater the mobility of the factors of production, the flatter the supply curve; and iii) the availability of stocks: where a product can be stored without loss of quality or undue expense, the supply curve will tend to be relatively flat. More on costs in Chapter 14.

The steepness of a demand curve shows the responsiveness of quantity demanded to changes in price. A relatively steep demand curve means that the

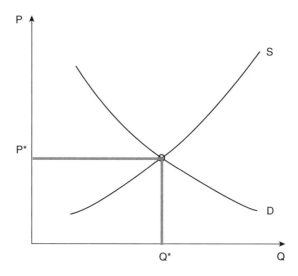

Fig. 2.12 Market equilibrium where supply equals demand.

quantity demanded is not very sensitive to the price of the good. A relatively flat demand curve means that the quantity demanded is sensitive to the price of the good. How sensitive the demand is to the price of the good is formulated in terms of a demand elasticity.

2.4.1 **Elasticities of demand**

The price elasticity of demand is the relative change in quantity, X, following a relative change in its own price, p_X:

$$\varepsilon = (\Delta X / X) / (\Delta p_X / p_X) \tag{2.7}$$

This elasticity is normally negative, because demand will fall when the price increases. The question is then by how much: If the quantity demanded changes relatively more than the price has changed, then demand is referred to as being elastic. Remember that since ε is negative, it follows that $\varepsilon < -1$. The higher its value (in absolute term), the more elastic the demand for a particular good, i.e. the more sensitive consumers are to its price. Such goods are of the kind we can easily live without if they become too expensive, or other similar goods ('substitutes', see below) exist that we would then choose instead.

If the quantity demanded changes relatively less than the price has changed ($\varepsilon > -1$), we say that demand is inelastic—illustrated by a steep demand curve. The smaller the value of the demand elasticity (again, in absolute terms), the less sensitive consumers are to its price. Such goods are needed more or less irrespective of their price, because there are few alternatives to them.

The above elasticity is more precisely referred to as own price elasticity, because it is the responsiveness of quantity demanded to changes in its own price—as opposed to price change of another good. More generally, the demand for good X is a function not only of its own price, p_X, as the two-dimensional Figure 2.12 might make us believe, but of (at least) two other important factors. These are the price of other goods, and income. For simplicity, the demand function (Equation 2.8) includes the price of only one other good, Y, and income, I:

$$D_X = f(p_X, p_Y, I) \tag{2.8}$$

When two goods X and Y are related to one another, changing the price of Y would impact upon the demand for X. This is referred to as cross price elasticity of demand ε_C:

$$\varepsilon_C = (\Delta X / X) / (\Delta p_Y / p_Y) \tag{2.9}$$

If two goods are positively related to one another, in that more of X also implies more of Y, they are referred to as complementary goods. A UK example might be gin and tonic, a Norwegian one is skis and ski poles. Goods are defined as complementary when the cross price elasticity is negative, e.g. when the price of gin increases, the demand for tonic falls. If two goods are negatively related to each other, they are referred as substitute goods. A US example of close substitutes is Pepsi-Cola and Coca-Cola. Goods are defined as substitutes when the cross price elasticity is positive, e.g. when the price of Pepsi increases relative to that of Coca-Cola, the demand for Coca-Cola increases.

The final type of elasticity to be introduced here is income elasticity, ε_I, i.e. relative increased demand following a relative income increase:

$$\varepsilon_I = (\Delta X / X) / (\Delta I / I) \tag{2.10}$$

Goods are referred to as normal goods when demand increases as income increases, i.e. the income elasticity is positive. If demand increases relatively less than income increases, the good is labelled a necessity ($\varepsilon_I < 1$), as opposed to a luxury, which is a good whose demand increases relatively more than the income increase ($\varepsilon_I > 1$).[1]

---

[1] An Oxfam advertisement in the UK was intended to draw attention to the fact that—to some people in the world—even the most basic necessity may feel like a luxury: 'Everybody deserves life's little luxuries: you know, food, water, that sort of thing.'

When the above elasticities are being calculated, all variables in the demand function are held constant except the determining factor. It is the isolated impact of this factor that is being measured.

In a health policy context, these elasticities would be helpful for answering a range of public health issues. An own price elasticity is required to answer: how much reduction in the demand for cigarettes can be expected from a given increase in tobacco taxation? A cross price elasticity is required to answer: how much increased demand for marijuana can be expected (e.g. among 16–20-year-olds) by a given price increase on beer? An income elasticity is required to answer: how much increased demand for private health insurance can be expected after a given increase in income?

As well as movements up and down particular demand and supply curves, we can also consider shifts in the curves. A shift in the demand curve would be caused by a change in other parameters in the demand function besides price. For example, higher incomes tend to shift the demand curve further out. The curve would also shift out when suppliers (perhaps through advertising) persuade consumers that the good is even better or even more needed than consumers had originally thought. In health economics, the concept of supplier-induced demand is illustrated by such shifts in the demand curve—here, demand is induced by doctors who recommend that patients use more health care (see Chapter 10). A shift in the supply curve is typically caused by technological changes, whereby marginal costs change—e.g. technological innovation—would make the supply curve shift downwards. All exogenous shifts in the demand or supply curve result in a new equilibrium price and output.

Demand for health care

As with all other goods, the demand function for health care includes not only the price of health care, but many other variables: *income* (the richer you are, the more are you able to pay), *distance* to health care providers (the further away you live, the higher your 'time costs' and hence the less you demand), and *provider behaviour* (if the doctor has few patients on their list, they may recommend you to demand more). While these other factors are important determinants of the observed demand for health care, they are easily forgotten when focusing on a demand curve that shows how demand varies with the magnitude of patient charges *only*.

Probably the most important insight into the study of demand for health care is that this reflects a *derived demand for health* (Grossman, 1972). It is not health care per se that people demand, but rather improved health. Thus, we demand health care for its expected effect on our health.

The concept of efficiency in a nutshell

Technical efficiency: all points on the isoquant

Technical efficiency is the first level of efficiency and refers to all combinations of input factors *on* the isoquant. This means that we do not waste scarce resources. Points to the north-east of the isoquant involve using more input factors than necessary, i.e. a waste of resources.

Cost efficiency: the cheapest combination on the isoquant

When all points on the isoquant are technically efficient, *which* one should we choose? Choose the point that is tangential to a budget line, because that is the cheapest combination of inputs. This second level of efficiency is referred to as *cost efficiency*. The exact point chosen on the isoquant will depend on the relative prices of the input factors.

Pareto-efficiency in production

The production possibility frontier (PPF) helps to explain efficiency regarding which *combination of two goods* should be produced. It shows the maximum alternative combinations of two goods that can be produced given the total available input factors. The collection of frontier points is referred to as being *Pareto-efficient*. This means that at any point on the frontier it is not possible to increase the production of X without reducing the production of Y. The rate at which this can be done is given by the marginal rate of transformation between X and Y (MRT_{XY}). Clearly, points inside the frontier cannot be Pareto-efficient.

Allocative efficiency: the preferred combination of goods

When all points on the PPF are referred to as being Pareto-efficient in production, *which* point on the PPF should be chosen? The answer is the combination of the goods which corresponds with consumer preferences, i.e. where the consumer's marginal rate of substitution between X and Y (MRS_{XY}) is equal to the MRT_{XY}. At this point, the factors of production have been allocated between the production of the two goods so as to reflect what people demand. This unique combination of the two goods corresponds with allocative efficiency.

The concept of efficiency in a nutshell–(continued)

An important reminder: allocative efficiency crucially depends on the policy objective

In the above standard definition of allocative efficiency following from neo-classical welfare economics, it is implicitly (sometimes explicitly) assumed that social welfare is a function of individual utilities, signalled through willingness to pay. This maximand is quite contentious in the context of health care, where an alternative welfare function, or maximand, is often explicitly stated as maximizing population health. Allocative efficiency would then refer to the point on the 'health possibility frontier' that involves the highest total health (see Chapter 4).

2.5 Conclusion

The equilibrium point at which demand equals supply offers an attractive theoretical solution to 'the grand economic problem' of how much to produce in order to maximize welfare. The interaction between producers and consumers, each of them acting out of their own self-interest, brings about an optimal outcome where social welfare is maximized. The idea that an 'invisible hand' can bring about allocative efficiency has been immensely attractive to economists since the founding father of modern economics, Adam Smith (1723–1790), introduced this parable. However, the 'invisible hand' is troublesome in the real world where a range of restrictive assumptions will have to be satisfied for the market to be the ideal system for achieving efficiency. The next chapter sets out these assumptions, and discusses market failures that are of particular relevance to health care.

Suggested reading

An introductory economics text: Begg, D., Fischer, S. and Dornbusch, R. (2003) *Economics*. London: McGraw-Hill.

A somewhat more advanced text in microeconomics: Varian, H. (2005) *Intermediate Microeconomics: A Modern Approach*. London: W. W. Norton.

Exercises

1. Return to Table 2.3 and the figure you drew in relation to it. Compute the total costs of the different combinations when an employee costs $400 and a machine costs $200 per day. What is then the cheapest (i.e. the most cost effective) combination of L and K?

2. Explain the difference between *average* productivity and *marginal* productivity. Why is this difference important to decision makers? Give a numerical example.

3. Explain to a friend or colleague what is meant by *cost* efficiency and *allocative* efficiency. Use examples from the health service.

Chapter 3

What makes the market for health care different?

Public intervention in the market for health care is based on two quite separate reasons: 'market failures' and equity. This chapter explores the nature of market failures, emphasizing the *efficiency* reasons for regulating health care markets.

The specific characteristics of the market for health care will be analysed with reference to the general model of the perfectly competitive market. The context of this inquiry into 'failures' follows the neoclassical economic tradition, where benefits are assessed and valued by consumer preferences as these are expressed by their willingness to pay. If, on the contrary, benefits are to be valued in terms of health improvements and health care is to be distributed in accordance with the principle of 'equal access for equal need', there are *equity* reasons for intervening in health care markets—a topic for Chapter 4.

3.1 The perfect market model and the imperfect market for health care

A market can be defined as any place where the sellers of a particular good or service can meet with the buyers of that good and service, where there is a potential for a transaction to take place. Such meeting points for transaction and trading could be anything from an old village market to a supermarket or an online marketplace such as eBay.

A distinguishing feature in economic theories of markets is the number of sellers. If there is one seller only, that is referred to as a monopoly; if there are two sellers, it is a duopoly; and if there is a handful or more, it is referred to as an oligopoly. In these types of markets sellers are able to charge higher prices for their goods than the cost of producing them. Such markets would therefore not be considered perfect for consumers. A key characteristic of what economists refer to as a *perfect* market, or a perfectly competitive market, is one in which there is such a large number of sellers that none of them is able to influence the price.

The perfectly competitive market is a very attractive mechanism for distributing goods and services: consumers get what they want if they pay what things cost, and producers get sufficient revenues to cover their costs. Due to the harsh competition between producers, any profits over and above what is needed to keep them in business evaporate in the long run. The market clearing point—or the equilibrium—in which supply equals demand (look back at Figure 2.12) yields a market *price* where the marginal social value equals the marginal social costs, and the *quantity* produced equals the quantity demanded.

Beyond serving as an attractive model, the perfectly competitive market also serves as a yardstick against which the imperfect real world can be compared with an ideal model world. But what is required for a market to be *perfect*?

To understand why real markets do not always operate so perfectly, Table 3.1 sets out the fairly restrictive assumptions upon which the perfect market model rests.

Even the most 'pro-market' economists admit that not many real world markets satisfy *all* of the above assumptions completely. However, the reason

Table 3.1 Some key assumptions behind the perfect market model

Assumption	Implication
1. Full information	Buyers know how much and when they wish to consume, as well as the quality of the goods.
2. Impersonal transactions	Buyers and sellers act independently and operate at 'arm's length'.
3. Private goods	Only the person consuming the good is affected by it; they pay all the social costs and gain all the social benefits.
4. Selfish motivation	Buyers are 'only in it for getting satisfaction', and sellers are 'only in it for the profit'.
5. Many buyers and sellers	No single buyer or seller can influence the market price, neither alone nor through coordinated action.
6. Free entry (and exit)	Anyone who would like to sell the products may start to do so, and anyone may leave the market whenever they want.
7. Homogeneous products	Buyers cannot distinguish between the products of the different producers.

why 'imperfect' markets may still be favoured is that they are believed to work better than an alternative with public regulation and public ownership. We can think of real world markets located on a spectrum ranging from (almost) *perfect* to (almost) *imperfect*. The market for health care stands out as being almost completely imperfect. To what extent, then, are which of the assumptions in Table 3.1 not met in the market for health care?

The first assumption, of *full information*, consists of two separate issues: i) buyers can predict how much they want to buy and when, i.e. there is no *uncertainty* involved, and ii) buyers know the quality of the good, either through own experience from previous consumption or availability of *product information*.

The distinction between these two issues is important in the context of health care. First, individuals do not have *full information* about the timing or costs of illness. This means that planning expenditure on health care, even over a relatively short time period, is almost impossible. This gives rise to insurance markets and an associated set of market failures (see Chapters 7 and 8). Patients also lack information about the quality of health care and about the expected effect of health care on health: this is essentially why they see doctors in the first place. Of course, doctors are not fully informed either, but what is important here is that patients have much less information *relative* to doctors. This problem of asymmetric information between doctors (as providers or sellers) and patients (as consumers) is elaborated in section 3.2 below.

The assumption of *impersonal transactions* requires that buyers have the same level of trust and confidence in all sellers. They are completely indifferent as to who the seller is.

For many health care services, especially in primary care, buyers know who the producer is. The transactions between buyers and sellers are personal and their relationship will be based largely on trust. Thus, the notion of *impersonal transactions* between atomistic agents is not an appropriate description of the doctor—patient relationship, which is discussed more fully below. Interestingly, the rationale behind capitation payment in general practice is to encourage patients to stick to *one* general practitioner rather than shop around.

Private goods are goods where *only* the person consuming the good is affected by it. *Public goods* are different in that they can be jointly consumed by many people. Public goods are characterized by: i) *non-rivalry*, i.e. the consumption of the good by one person does not preclude its consumption by another person (e.g. street lights), and ii) *non-excludability*, i.e. individuals can receive the benefits of a good without having to pay for it. When users do not have an incentive to pay for public goods, such goods are under-provided.

Some preventive health programmes targeted at those environmental factors that impact on people's health can be conceived of as 'public goods', e.g. reduction of toxic air pollution, and malarial control such as pond clearing. These programmes are characterized by non-rivalry in that everybody in the community will benefit from clean air without stopping anyone else from benefiting. Additionally, one cannot exclude those people in the community from benefiting who have not paid for its provision.

Somewhere in between pure *private goods* and pure *public goods* lie goods for which more people than the person consuming the good are being affected by it. Economists talk about *externalities* in consumption when there are 'by-product consequences'—which are *not* being priced in a market—on other people's utilities beyond the person making the consumption decision. When one person's consumption positively affects another person's utility we have a *positive externality*, e.g. putting the heat on in your flat may increase the temperature in the flat above you. The most typical example of a *negative externality* is smoking.

The economic problem with externalities is one of inefficiency. An unregulated market will under-provide goods with positive externalities, while it will over-provide goods with negative externalities. The standard market solution to the problem of externalities is to *internalize* them, i.e. make the person who consumes a good that includes externalities take into account its effects on others. Negative externalities should be *taxed* in accordance with the extra costs imposed on others, while positive externalities should be *subsidized* in accordance with the value of the extra benefits experienced by others. Some types of health care clearly involve positive externalities, which will be elaborated in section 3.3 below.

Selfish motivation may not necessarily govern people in all walks of life (fortunately), but it makes sense for describing much of our behaviour in the marketplace. Consumers buy goods simply because goods yield utility. Producers sell goods in order to make a profit.

Consumers and producers appear to behave quite differently in the market for health care. Patients may not be so selfish that they disregard any concern with how their condition impacts upon other people. And rarely, if ever, would doctors say that they practise medicine to maximize profits; even if they did, a code of professional ethics attempts to restrict them from doing so.

With *many buyers and sellers*, no single actor can influence the market price; we become 'price takers' in that we face a market price which results from uncoordinated actions.

There are certainly many buyers of health care, and in most cases they operate sufficiently independently of one another. The numbers of independent sellers will vary. Only in big cities would we find many hospitals, but general practitioners and specialists might be found in large numbers and may compete with each other in attracting patients. Overall, however, as judged from the assumption of many sellers and buyers, the market for health care is imperfect.

Whilst oligopolies (few sellers) and monopolies (one seller) are not unusual features of a market economy (where a few sellers may benefit from economies of scale and thus promote efficiency), economic theory considers competition to be good and monopoly to be bad. Monopolistic conditions will result in so-called *X inefficiencies* (such as managerial slack) due to the lack of incentive to produce at lowest cost, i.e. monopolies use more input factors than are necessary for a given output, and they are able to charge higher prices than would reflect marginal costs.

Free entry of health care providers is not a common feature of this market. There are professional regulations that prohibit non-medics from offering their services. In addition, certain types of professional qualifications are required in most countries for practitioners to receive public funding (e.g. physiotherapists). And even if they might be prepared to rely on patient payments, many countries regulate the number of various practitioners in any region. However, as in most markets, there is free exit in that doctors may stop practising whenever they want.

There may well be market conditions that prevent competition *in* the market (for example, economies of scale, which mean that technical efficiency is achieved through a sole supplier—a natural monopoly), but the idea is to create competition *for* the market. For contracting to work, the bidding environment must be competitive. This does not mean that the market itself has to be competitive. Provided that at least two bidders can offer to produce a specified service, and provided that the incumbent hospital (or its management) cannot ignore the threat of entry without risking being replaced by a new producer, then a competitive price and output will result. In other words, the market must be *contestable*. Successful contracting also requires a system whereby bidders' offers can be evaluated—and this requires information.

Clearly, if buyers can distinguish between products from different producers, they might develop a preference for one product over another, and hence be willing to pay more for it. It is quite a common market strategy for providers to attempt to make their products distinguishable from those of their competitors: a practice known as *product differentiation*.

The same goes for health care. Although the chemical substance of a drug from different producers may be *homogeneous*, drugs have brand names, and new and expensive drugs are claimed to be better. Private hospitals and physicians also attempt to make patients believe their services are of a higher quality than those of public providers by wrapping their services in more attractive amenities. Indeed, non-price competition is only possible if patients perceive the services provided by different hospitals or doctors to be different.

So, none of the seven assumptions listed in Table 3.1 would hold for describing health care markets in general. While some of these assumptions are not satisfied in many other markets either, the market for health care is distinguished by three key characteristics, according to Evans (1984). These are: i) uncertainty, ii) asymmetric information (i.e. the two violations of the assumption of full information), and iii) externalities. In addition to the 'selfish externalities' related to the fact that one person's health may affect other people's health or wealth, there is the so-called 'caring externality' in health, which refers to the altruistic reasons for subsidizing our fellow citizens' health care consumption.

The solution to uncertainty is insurance, which will be analysed in Chapters 7 and 8. The solution to asymmetric information is regulation of providers, which will be dealt with below, as well as in Chapters 10 and 11. The solution to externalities would primarily be various types of regulation and subsidization, which will be dealt with in section 3.3 below and in Chapter 4.

3.2 Asymmetric information and the agency relationship

Asymmetric information exists when one party possesses more information than the other, and where this information is of a kind that is considered important to the latter. Doctors possess two types of information that are important to patients: *diagnostic* information ('what is wrong with the patient?') and *treatment* information ('what can be done for the patient?'). As a consequence, a patient would want their doctor to act as their *perfect agent*. In general terms, an agency relationship exists when one individual or group (the agent) acts on behalf of another individual or group (the principal). We can consider a doctor as acting as an agent in two distinct ways. First, when he acts solely for an individual patient, and second, when he considers other people alongside that patient. For example, he might simultaneously consider his other patients or possibly a third-party payer, such as the government or society as a whole.

3.2.1 The doctor—patient relationship

The consumption of health care is different from the consumption of most other goods in that the consumer lacks information about the effects that health care will have on their utility. Unlike normal goods that are consumed for their direct utility-yielding properties, health care is consumed for its impact on health. Health care itself is not a 'good' in the conventional sense, but a 'bad' (or a necessary evil) required for improved health. Hence, the demand for health care is a *derived demand* for health. As with most other goods in the utility function, the individual is the best judge of their utility from health. Going back to Figure 1.2, the consumer is sovereign in judging the utility they get from health directly, as well as indirectly via the impact that health has on wealth and social relations.

However—and this is crucial—the consumer lacks information about the impact of health care on health, i.e. about the production function: $H = f(HC)$. Typically, the patient will lack information about which treatments might be available, and the effectiveness of the alternative treatments. On the other hand, the supplier of health care—the doctor—has much greater knowledge concerning the relationship between health care and health. Given this information asymmetry, it is not surprising that patients would prefer that doctors make decisions on their behalf.

Doctors do, however, differ in their views about what it is that patients want from them: some argue that their task is to tell the patient what treatment they should have, others that it is their task to provide the patient with information so that the patient can decide. *In theory*, this agency relationship is not a problem because the utility function of the agent (the doctor) is identical to that of the principal (the patient): that of maximizing the utility of each patient. As Williams (1988) points out, if the doctor is the perfect agent, 'The *doctor* is there to give the *patient* all the information the *patient* needs in order that the *patient* can make a decision, and the *doctor* should then implement that decision once the *patient* has made it.'

However, even if patients' and doctors' utility functions were identical (which is unlikely), this still requires that each doctor will have full knowledge of the arguments in each patient's utility function. Now, it seems reasonable to assume that maximizing health will be an objective of most patients. However, other arguments such as the amount of information requested or the desired degree of involvement in the decision-making process are likely to be important and will naturally differ across patients. Thus it is unlikely that any doctor could act as a perfect agent for their patient.

In reality, the agency relationship that has evolved in health care is one in which the supplier can greatly influence the consumer's utility function. Because doctors hold a position such that they can have some influence over both the costs and benefits of health care, there is the potential for exploitation. Williams (1988) claims that the more recognizable form of his characterization of the agency relationship is one in which the words 'doctor' and 'patient' are reversed: 'The *patient* is there to give the *doctor* all the information the *doctor* needs in order that the *doctor* can make a decision, and the *patient* should then implement that decision once the *doctor* has made it.'

It seems that the only effective constraints on the doctor's behaviour are medical ethics, which provide some reassurances that the doctor will attempt to do their best for the individual patient, and clinical guidelines, which aim to reduce the wide differences in medical practice. However, because the choice of treatment recommended by the 'seller' may have many important consequences for the 'buyer', the latter is better described as a vulnerable patient rather than an empowered consumer. So the market for health care clearly violates the assumption of impersonal market transactions: buyers and sellers are almost hugging one another rather than operating at arm's length. And because the doctor—patient relationship is so heavily based on trust, the doctor could exploit the patient in a variety of ways, possibly even inducing demand that might not otherwise exist (see Chapter 10).

3.2.2 **The agency relationship and social welfare**

Discussions of the individual doctor—patient relationship appear to suggest that a perfect agent is a doctor who provides the patient with the combination of services which is most preferred by the patient. However, what the patient wants might differ from what society wants. This raises questions about who the doctor is ultimately the agent for: the patient, a group of patients, health care funders, or society as a whole? Doctors, like the rest of us, cannot please all of the people all of the time, and so the answers to these question will determine what the perfect agent looks like.

Consider the following framework which, following the medical code of ethics that 'the health of my patient shall be my first consideration', is based on the assumption that doctors should act in the best interest of the patients ex post. This is against a background that the funders of health care may have two sets of preferences: one about the services they would like for themselves should they become ill, and one about those services that they are prepared to cross-subsidize for others. The idea comes from Evans (1984), who suggested that people might prefer complete discretion over their own care yet feel paternalistic about the care of others.

Within this framework, it can be shown that the size of the health care budget depends on the choices made by doctors regarding the mix they offer between health-enhancing services and those services that have no impact on health but which patients may still want for other utility-enhancing reasons.

If doctors provide a mix that reflects the preferences of patients ex post, funders will react by reducing their contributions to health care since they do not like to see health care being 'wasted' on services that do not improve health. However, the very same funders would still wish to see such services being available to themselves should they end up as patients.

Given such *split preferences*, doctors will act as perfect agents for their patients if they provide *fewer* non-health enhancing services than the very same patients would prefer. By restricting 'waste', the total health care budget is increased, thereby enabling doctors to treat more patients.[1] This model is based on an assumption that our willingness to cross-subsidize health care depends on the effectiveness of that care in improving health.

3.3 Externalities: selfishly motivated

Assuming that health care represents a private good would imply that nobody beyond the consumer/patient benefits from the use of health care. However, an inquiry into the various types of interpersonal relationships in health suggests that there are four different ways in which the improved health that a person obtains from their health care use may affect another person's utility. Externalities in the use of health care are illustrated in Figure 3.1, which represents an extension of Figure 1.2.

Figure 3.1 illustrates two individuals, A and B. The focus is on how B's improved health may affect A. Compared with Figure 1.2, the variable W, wealth, is subdivided into own consumption, C, and tax contributions, T, that go to finance government spending, G, i.e. public goods such as schools, parks, defence. Why would A care about B's use of health care (and vice versa, which for presentational reasons are not shown in this figure)? There are two *selfish* reasons that will be dealt with here, and two *altruistic* reasons that will be discussed in the next chapter.

The links illustrated in Figure 3.1, focusing on individual A's utility from his own utilization of health care, as well as indirectly via individual B's health (resulting from B's utilization of health care) can be formalized within an extended utility function (3.1):

$$U_A = u[SR_A, C_A, H_A(HC_A, H_B), G(H_A, H_B), H_B, U_B] \qquad (3.1)$$

In addition to A's own social relations, consumption, and health, there are *four partial links from B to A*: i) contagion H_A (H_B), ii) economic contributions

---

[1] For an elaboration of this model, see Clark and Olsen (1994).

HC = health care, H = health, C = consumption, T = tax, G = government spendings,
SR = social relations, U = utility

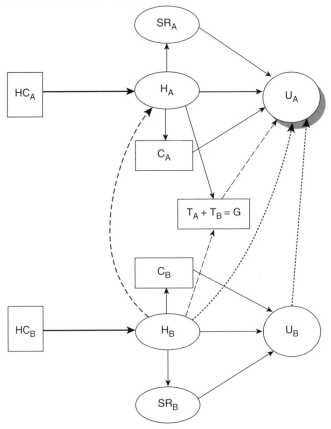

Fig. 3.1 The interpersonal relationships in health.

from B, G (H_B), iii) paternalistic altruism (caring for health) H_B, and iv)
general altruism (caring for general well-being) U_B.

3.3.1 **Contagion**

Contagion is illustrated in Figure 3.1 by the dotted arrow from H_B to H_A. This
refers to health care consumed by B that may have a positive impact on A's
health, such as vaccination and the cure of infectious diseases. In an unregulated market, B will consume this type of health care (like any other) up to the
level where the private benefits equal (social) costs. However, in a societal perspective, this is not sufficient due to the existence of *positive externalities*, which
imply that A (along with all other affected fellow members of society) will

experience benefits beyond B's individual benefits. These benefits—as valued by the rest of society—should be added to the individual benefits in order to derive *aggregate social benefits*.

So how can such market failures be corrected for; how can the externalities be internalized? The simple answer is for the rest of society to cross-subsidize B's costs of these services to the extent that B will face private costs so low that they will choose to consume the socially optimal quantity. To illustrate this, let us assume that an individual's private benefit (*PB*) is given by their maximum willingness to pay for health care. The external benefits (*EB*) are those that are valued by other people besides the consumer—through *their* willingness to pay. Therefore, the summation of *PB* and *EB* represents social benefits (*SB*). Let us also assume that all relevant social costs (*SC*) are included. The optimal amount consumed is where *SB* = *SC*:

$$PB + EB = SB = SC \tag{3.2}$$

The optimal level of cross-subsidization implies that *EB* is subtracted from *SC*. In Figure 3.2, *PB* illustrates the private demand curve, and *SB* represents society's demand curve. Thus, the vertical distance between the two curves reflects *EB*. For simplicity, we have assumed constant marginal *SC*. The intersection between *PB* and *SC* gives the private quantity, X_P, which is where the individual would choose to consume in the absence of any influence from others. The intersection between *SB* and *SC* gives the socially optimal quantity, X_S. The individual can be induced to move there if we subsidize health care by the vertical distance between *SB* and *PB* at this quantity.

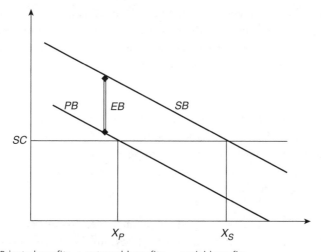

Fig. 3.2 Private benefits + external benefits = social benefits.

Interestingly, this optimal level of cross-subsidy (i.e. the vertical distance between the two benefit curves at the point where $SB = SC$) does *not* imply that consumers would face a zero price. Analytically, this represents a special case. Figure 3.2 illustrates an optimal solution where the consumer has to pay a positive amount. It is, however, quite possible to imagine situations where the external benefits to the rest of society might be so large that the locus of the intersection between SB and SC might even imply that individual consumers should face a *negative* private price; that is, they should be paid to consume health care (more on this in Chapter 10).

Any cross-subsidy could take the form of voluntary donations, tax financing, or through information campaigns. The growth of public health care is very much a history of fighting contagious diseases, and immunization and vaccination have at various times been mandatory (as well as provided free of charge, of course).

3.3.2 Economic contribution to society

An important consequence of improved health is that it affects people's productive capacity. Not surprisingly, economists have recognized for a long time the importance of healthy labour for economic growth. For example, the early economic evaluation techniques considered the increased value of production from improved health as the way to measure outcomes from treatments—the focus was on repairing an input factor, the human capital. This increased productivity would increase income, which in turn increases consumption. In an influential health economic model, these impacts are termed the 'investment benefits' from health, as opposed to the 'consumption benefits' that follow from the enjoyment of being in better health (Grossman, 1972).

If increased production ends up as own consumption only, and if we are indifferent to a fellow citizen's consumption level, then there are no externalities from the wealth generated. However, in most economies, some of the increase in an individual's wealth ends up contributing towards society, e.g. people pay income tax, which goes towards the financing of public goods and services. The self-interested reasons why we are concerned with our fellow citizens' increased economic contributions to society are, first, that public goods and services are positive arguments in our utility function, and second, if a sufficient level of such goods was already produced, then more contribution from others means that we will have to pay less ourselves.

Therefore, if the only reason why we care about the health of others were because of their economic contribution to society beyond their own consumption (the link in Figure 3.1 between $H_B \rightarrow T_B \rightarrow G \rightarrow U_A$), we would be willing to subsidize their health care so that they could return to the workforce. We would do so as long as the expected future economic contributions exceed the costs of treatment, i.e. as long as people 'pay their way' in terms of their use of collective resources ($T_B - HC_B > 0$).

The implication of this type of selfish concern for others is of course that we would provide a higher subsidy to those groups in society who will make the highest economic contributions from being treated. One way that this has been put into practice in some countries is to have sickness benefit funds that pay the costs of treating people who would return to work as a consequence of cure. While this may be a quite rational selfish argument, it might well be that there is a conflict here with one of the key equity objectives of many health systems; namely, 'equal access for equal need', independent of economic position.

3.4 **Conclusion**

No market works perfectly. But some work less perfectly than others—and the market for health care appears to be one of them. There are a number of reasons for market failure in health care and this chapter has highlighted the most pervasive. In essence, the market fails primarily because of a range of informational asymmetries.

There are a number of ways in which the market mechanism can be improved to mitigate the adverse consequences of various kinds of asymmetric information, but every country in the world recognizes the need for considerable government involvement and regulation in the market for health care. It is important to reiterate that this involvement and regulation could be motivated out of a concern for efficiency alone: we might not care one jot about equity and still have government involvement in health care. The discussion of externalities in this chapter has highlighted two of the most important efficiency-motivated responses to market failure. When we add equity and distributional considerations to the picture, the case for replacing the market mechanism in many parts of health care becomes overwhelming.

Suggested reading

A standard reference: Arrow, K. (1963) Uncertainly and the welfare economics of medical care. *American Economic Review*, 53, 941–73.

Evans, R. G. (1984) *Strained Mercy: The economics of Canadian health care*. Toronto: Butterworths (Chapters 2–4 analyse health care market failures brilliantly; available at http://www.chspr.ubc.ca/publications?type=6).

Exercises

1. The assumption of *full information* is not met in the market for health care. Explain its two distinctly different failures of *uncertainty* and *asymmetric information*.

2. Discuss various regulations of health care providers that are intended to protect patients.

3. Illustrate the situation in which external benefits exceed social costs: explain how we can achieve the socially optimal quantity.

Chapter 4

Equality and fairness

This chapter begins with an inquiry into altruism and redistribution before we explore the issues of equality and fairness as applied to the distribution of health and health care. Altruism is seen through the eyes of 'the individual as a consumer', while equity is seen through the eyes of 'the individual as a citizen'.

In the previous chapter, Figure 3.1 identified four types of interpersonal relationships in health, i.e. how the health of person B might affect the utility of person A. Two of these were labelled selfishly motivated externalities. The other two are of a more altruistic kind and will be discussed below.

4.1 Externalities: *un*selfishly motivated

Why does redistribution take place? The various explanations reflect different political ideologies. To libertarians, all redistribution (other than that based on individual voluntary donations) is *coerced*. They perceive the rich as being forced through the political process and the ballot box to redistribute some of their income to the poor who hold the political power due to the 'tyranny of the majority'. A Marxist explanation of redistribution would be to consider it as an insurance for the ruling capitalists, who will reduce the probability of revolution by bribing the working class with such things as a minimum income, pensions, and access to education and health care. These rather cynical explanations leave little room for people to care genuinely for one another: either the poor are seen as ripping off the rich, or the rich are seen as offering some minimum compensation in return for exploiting the poor.

The third explanation that we shall go into more closely is based on the view that people *care* about their fellow citizens. The idea of *voluntary* redistribution reflects this altruism and can be analysed within the framework of interdependent utility functions. Set within a two-person economy with a rich person, R, and a poor person, P, redistribution involves R giving away some of their income to P $(- \Delta Y_R = \Delta Y_P)$. Voluntary redistribution will continue until R's gain in marginal utility from P's increased income is equal to R's marginal utility loss from his own reduced income.

However, voluntary redistribution may lead to a lower degree of redistribution than that which would be considered optimal by rich people. One reason for this is 'free-riding', which may occur when we extend the model from a two-person to an n-person world. Here, a rich person could watch all their rich mates contribute towards the poor but, because the marginal benefit to the poor from the rich person's own contribution would be small, the rich person might not do likewise. In other words, this rich person could 'free-ride' on the backs of the contribution of others. So it may be rational for rich people to vote for compulsory redistributive taxation so that their mates do not free-ride. This offers an explanation of why rich citizens may opt for 'voluntary compulsion' and vote for political parties whose tax policies will reduce their own private consumption: an explanation that makes sense only when distinguishing between the individual as citizen and as consumer.

Still, this degree of voluntary redistribution (even when decided collectively among the rich to be made compulsory) will be optimal only so far as rich people are concerned. If the rest of the people in society (i.e. the poor) are of the opinion that it is fair for the rich to give away more, it follows that voluntary redistribution will produce less equality than that which would result from democratic majority rule.

Voluntary redistribution reflects some form of altruism, which is the opposite of selfishness. According to *The Concise Oxford Dictionary* (6th edition) altruism means 'regard for others as a principle of action'. However, actions that are basically to the benefit of others might also have a 'selfish side effect'. Equally, actions that are basically selfishly motivated might result in benefits to others. Why, then, do we care about other people and how do we identify actions that have purely selfless motivations?

A first set of explanations for altruism is that the donor gets personal utility from showing sympathy or undertaking actions that they consider to be social duties. In other words, donors 'purchase moral satisfaction' or get 'warm glow' feelings from doing good things. So, in order to obtain a feeling of being a decent citizen, the donor is motivated to act in ways that benefit others. The father of economics, Adam Smith, has been widely quoted as championing self-interest, but this is a mistaken view. Despite recognizing that 'self-love' enabled mutually advantageous trade to take place, he did not assign a generally superior role to the pursuit of self-interest. However, much of Smith's writings on the role of ethical considerations in human behaviour have become neglected as these considerations have become unfashionable in economics.

Certainly some types of actions that might appear to be altruistic are not so. One type can be explained by *reciprocity*, that is, we do good things for others because we hope and expect that they will do the same in return. This is the mentality of 'I'll scratch your back, if you scratch mine,' i.e. I depend on someone else to do something I appreciate (scratch my back), and the price I pay is to do the same thing for that person.

While this example deals with one-to-one reciprocity, the idea of reciprocity can be extended to society, i.e. I'll do good things for others because I might rely on my fellow citizens doing good things for me. Such reciprocity might be seen as investment and insurance for the purposes of creating a supportive social climate that is to the benefit of all, i.e. a climate of *solidarity*. And in this sense, reciprocity is motivated from concerns other than the direct personal utility from giving per se.

Another type of action that might appear to be altruistic is what we refer to as '*conspicuous altruism*'. This is inspired by the concept of 'conspicuous consumption' which refers to how higher socio-economic groups use some types of consumption as a means of showing off their excess wealth.[1] The foremost aim of this type of consumption is to signal a successful social position. Analogous to the concept of purchasing moral satisfaction, people can purchase social approval through conspicuous altruism. This might acquire even greater social status in that donors are seen as doing something good for others rather than as spending excess wealth on frivolous private consumption. The rationale behind making donations conspicuous, then, is that the donors know that they can be identified by society, which will bestow social approval on them.

Some types of actions that benefit others might be to the direct benefit of oneself. Other actions, whose *outcomes* are clearly to the benefit of others, might be influenced by selfishness in the *process* of giving. When we say that we care for the health or well-being of known individuals who are part of our social relations, such as family and friends, this might be explained by the fact that we are directly affected by their suffering. Being affected could involve constraints on our own life (e.g. caring for a sick child) or could simply result

---

[1] A concept introduced by the Norwegian-American economist and sociologist Thorstein Veblen (1857–1929).

in our being emotionally stressed. We resist using the term altruism when there is such direct benefit.

Is anything left that we can legitimately call *genuine* altruism? To qualify as genuine altruism an action must by way of motivation not contain any degree of reciprocity; it should not involve any element of gaining social approval; and the donor cannot have any personal or social relations with the beneficiaries. Genuine altruism exists when we simply care that other people's well-being has fallen below a level that we consider to be acceptable. Rich and fit people may be observed to care for poor and sick ones. Looking back at Figure 3.1, we note two altruistic arrows, indicating that individual A may care for the health of individual B ($H_B \rightarrow U_A$) and/or for B's utility or well-being ($U_B \rightarrow U_A$). The former suggests that subsidies should be in the form of health care while the latter suggests cash transfers.

4.2 **Transfers in cash or in kind**

There is a spectrum from *general altruism* to *paternalistic altruism* defined according to the extent to which the donor respects the preferences of the recipient. At one extreme lies general altruism which, consistent with the new welfare economics, regards each individual as the best judge of their own welfare. In such cases, the donor is happy for the recipient to do whatever they like with the redistributed income. A transfer in cash will then allow the recipient to maximize their utility. At the other extreme lies paternalistic, or goods-focused, altruism. This involves limiting or changing the choice set of the recipient, usually in line with the preference of the donor.

Consider the following example of a donor's choice of a present, the money size of which is constrained by the cost of a compact disc (CD). If a general altruist, the donor would hand over the cash, which the recipient could then spend on anything. A goods-focused altruist, on the other hand, might buy the recipient a particular CD that they ('the pater') thinks the recipient *ought to* listen to. Of course, there are weaker forms of paternalistic altruism. For example, the donor might buy a gift voucher for the type of music they feel the recipient should listen to (e.g. in a classical CD shop). Or alternatively, and closer to the general altruist, the donor might simply feel that the recipient should consume music (of whatever style) and hence might buy a gift voucher from a general CD shop.

It is worth noting here that limiting the choice set of the recipient does not necessarily have to be line with the preferences of the donor. It might well be in accordance with the recipient's best interests as judged by some third party. For instance, we might know that pension savings, education, nutrition, housing and access to health care are all goods that we would like to have available to us. In this sense, such transfers are in accordance with the long-term interests of the recipient. However, it is paternalistic insofar as it involves limiting the *immediate* choice set of the consumer. In the behavioural economics literature, this type of paternalism is referred to as 'soft paternalism', which refers to the view that the state can help you make the choices you would make for yourself, if only you had the strength of will. Unlike 'hard paternalism', the softer kind aims only to skew your decisions in accordance with your long-term interest.

The extended utility function set out in Equation 3.1 contained a set of 'selfish attributes' (own social relations, own consumption, own health, public goods), and two types of altruism: i) paternalistic, or goods-focused, altruism (caring for health), and ii) general altruism (caring for general well-being).

A's paternalism towards the health of B could be explained by A's preference that B should live a healthy lifestyle. Or it might be that A views B's health as instrumental to B's ability to 'flourish' as a human being. So ultimately A is concerned with B's well-being but believes health is central to that. In either case, A has a stronger preference for health relative to other goods than A thinks B has.

A standard model in economics textbooks is to explain why—in terms of the recipient's utility—transfers in cash are always better than transfers in kind. This should be intuitively obvious: if the money value of an in-kind transfer were handed over as a cash transfer, the recipient can acquire the same in-kind bundle if that is what they want. However, if they choose to spend some or all of the money on other goods, then this reveals that they get higher utility from an alternative consumption bundle. Thus, in those cases where the recipient would not choose to spend all of their cash transfers on the good that would otherwise be transferred in kind, a smaller transfer in cash than in kind is required to bring about a given increase in utility.

This 'proof' in favour of cash transfers is based upon an implicit assumption that the donor is a general altruist, i.e. the size of the donation is independent of what the recipient spends the transfer on. However, one of the main reasons for in-kind transfers is that the donor (or some third party acting on their behalf) believes that some goods are more important to the recipient's well-being than other goods—and that, when left to their devices, the recipient will go for other goods (which are 'less good' in the eyes of the donor). If the donor's contribution would be lower if the transfer is in cash rather than in kind (because they are paternalistic), then the recipient might in fact gain greater utility from a larger in-kind transfer than from a smaller cash one.

Economics textbooks often refer to the type of goods that are being transferred in kind as 'merit goods', i.e. goods in respect of which the state overrides consumer preferences.[2] This concept is often extended to distinguish between 'merit goods' and 'demerit goods' (or 'merit bads'), where the consumption of the former is believed to be good for people and should therefore be subsidized, while consumption of the latter is believed to be bad for people and should therefore be restricted or taxed.

The problem with the concept of merit goods (and bads) is that the justification for overriding consumer preferences is unclear. As suggested above, it would seem to be indicative of the morality of the donors or a reflection of a genuine concern for the long-term interest of the recipient, and these are sometimes very difficult to disentangle. There are many economists, philosophers—and lay persons—who possess the rhetorical skills of presenting their own moral beliefs and prejudices as being consistent with the best interests of other people. In any event, the rationale behind transfers in kind is to limit the choice set of recipients, so as to encourage the consumption of goods or discourage the consumption of bads. The provision of specific health services, rather than providing people with health 'vouchers' which they might then trade on the open or black markets, certainly limits their choices.

Once the preferences of paternalistic donors are included in the calculation of social welfare along with the preferences of recipients, there is a tension between preserving a central tenet of welfare economics that each individual is the best judge of their own welfare and adopting a position which allows the preferences of the donors—in regard to recipients' well-being—to dominate. Much of the debate between the 'welfarist' and the 'non-welfarist' (or 'extra-welfarist') paradigm in economics revolves around this tension.

Within the bundle of merit goods, some will undoubtedly be considered to be more meritorious than others. While health care in general is referred to as a 'merit good', some types of health care are clearly more important in the eyes of the subsidizer. The observed differences in society's willingness to subsidize various types of health care might be explained by different degrees of paternalistic altruism.

So far, caring and sharing have been considered in the context of an individual utility function – in a two-person economy with rich, R, and poor, P. Let us now extend to consider a three-person economy with one rich, R, and two poor persons, P_1 and P_2, in which the rich person cares for the *health* of

[2] The concept was introduced by the American economist Richard Musgrave (1910–2007).

their fellow citizens, i.e. R is a paternalistic altruist. Equation 3.1 can then be revised and simplified to:

$$U_R = u(SR_R, C_R, H_R, G, H_{P1}, H_{P2}) \tag{4.1}$$

So who does R have the greatest altruistic concerns for, P_1 or P_2? If they are equal in all relevant aspects, it is difficult to imagine that R should feel more altruism for one over the other. Hence, R would most likely divide their health care subsidies equally between them: 'equals are to be treated equally'.

While it is fruitful to discuss altruism towards other citizens within the framework of an individual utility function, this framework makes less sense for discussing preferences over equity principles that include the whole of society. We will therefore move away from the preferences of the individual as a consumer and towards their preferences as a citizen. As a private individual, they are motivated by personal utility, and as a citizen, they are motivated by the utility of the collective. Harsanyi (1955) has suggested that an individual has two sets of preferences—one based on what they personally prefer and one relating to social considerations—that may come into conflict with one another.

4.3 Three theories of distributive justice

There are three theories of distributive justice that have particular relevance in the context of fairness in the allocation of health care. In their origin, these theories have different views regarding which entities are to be distributed, i.e. what the 'distribuendum' is. Still, they are perfectly applicable for analysing and comparing different preferred distributions when health is the distribuendum.

4.3.1 Utilitarianism

Defining an individual's welfare in terms of the utility (or happiness) they derive owes much to the work of the utilitarian philosophers, Jeremy Bentham (1748–1832) and John Stuart Mill (1806–1873). The original hedonistic perspective of Bentham is based on the simple premise that people do things to attain pleasure and to avoid pain. He believed that pleasure promotion and pain avoidance could be measured cardinally as a number of *utils*, which could then be used to make interpersonal comparisons, and thus provide information regarding how happy one person is compared with another.

Bentham was neutral about the sources of pleasure and pain: it is for each individual to decide these things for themselves. Mill, however, distinguished between 'higher' and 'lower' pleasures, famously claiming, 'It is better to be a human being dissatisfied than a pig satisfied; better to be Socrates dissatisfied than a fool satisfied.' The view that some types of consumption patterns are more approved of than others implies that society should *weight* pleasures in accordance with them being of a 'higher' or a 'lower' order.

From Mill onwards, utilitarian philosophers have shown increasing interest in the *source* of an individual's utility. Although a fully informed rational person is still taken to be the best judge of their own welfare, recent models do allow for preferences to be 'laundered' in various ways. This might be to correct them for mistaken beliefs or to allow for the exclusion of certain antisocial preferences. Therefore, whilst the distribuendum in a utilitarian framework is obviously still utility, it is far from obvious *what types* of utility should be allowed to contribute towards social welfare.

Utilitarian models do, however, rely on an individual's subjective assessment of their own utility. The crucial distributional issue is how many utils one individual is capable of generating from the consumption of an additional unit of a good compared with how many utils another individual is capable of generating from the same unit.

The *reason* why one individual may obtain more utility than another individual from a particular good consumed is not an issue: one individual may have different needs or one may just simply be a more effective 'pleasure generating machine', i.e. easier to please. But there are circumstances (for example, when deciding whether or not to give money to a beggar) where we will make our decision based upon what we think the person 'needs' rather on what they want. In this way, we may feel obliged to feed a beggar but not to finance his gambling.

The utilitarian philosophy aggregates utility across individuals according to an unweighted *sum-ranking rule*; that is, it looks only at the sum total of utilities, justified by 'the greatest happiness principle'. As a result, even the tiniest gain in the total sum would be taken to outweigh distributional inequalities of the most blatant kind. However, it is worth remembering that Bentham was in favour of radical redistribution: to argue that each person counted for only one in 18th-century Britain was radical indeed. If it is assumed that there is diminishing marginal utility of income, then redistribution from rich to poor will bring about a gain in the sum total of utilities. Note, however, that this concern for distribution is not part of the aggregation rule as such but rather comes from assumptions that are made about the shape of an individual's utility function (Figure 2.2).

Utilitarianism appears in a modified and simplified version when maximizing health. Rather than utility or happiness, health is the maximand, and the utilitarian 'greatest happiness principle' is thus being translated to 'the greatest (total) health principle'. Health maximization is a much simpler principle to implement in policy practice than utility maximization: first, as opposed to the measurement of utility, there are widely accepted methods for cardinal measurement of health states; second, individual differences in relative strengths of preferences for health are disregarded by assigning the same finite end points (0–1) on the cardinal health scale; and third, interpersonal comparisons of health gains are made from the normative judgement that a given health gain is assigned the same social value irrespective of the characteristics of the patients involved.

4.3.2 **Egalitarianism**

The term *general* egalitarianism is often used when the distribuendum is income or wealth, whilst *specific* egalitarianism refers to the view that there ought to be an equal distribution of a particular good. However, independently of whether it is general or specific, egalitarianism is referred to as being 'strong' when the preferred solution is the one with the most equal distribution of the distribuendum. Strong egalitarianism can be distinguished from the egalitarianism of maximin that allows for inequalities so long as they benefit the worst off (see section below). For example, strong egalitarians would prefer an equal split of 50 units (of utility, primary goods, health, etc.) to each of two individuals to a situation where one individual had 80 and the other 51. This is because the latter situation is more unequal (80 / 51) than the former (50 / 50), even though the worst-off individual would benefit from having 51 rather than 50.

Elster (1992) refers to strong egalitarianism as 'strongly envious'. Whilst it may represent an extreme distribution rule, it is not absurd and does not have to be explained by envy. For example, children often instinctively interpret justice as synonymous with absolute equality. Reinhardt (1998) provides a great example of bringing home chocolate bars to two siblings, where clearly a Pareto-inferior combination (2 / 2) is better (in terms of peace and harmony) than a combination (3 / 4) that adheres to the assumption of monotonicity ('more is better').

However, when the distribuendum is no longer income but health, strong egalitarianism would be absurd in a policy context. It suggests that a situation in which two individuals are in an equally bad state of health is considered better than the situation in which only one is in that state and the other is fit and healthy. Hence, at least in the context of health, we believe maximin emerges as a more sensible rule than strong egalitarianism.

4.3.3 **Maximin**

In his theory of justice, John Rawls (1921–2002) is egalitarian at the outset, but accepts inequality as long as it is not possible to further the improvement of the worst off. Rawls (1971) held that 'social and economic inequalities must be to the greatest benefit of the least advantaged'. This he refers to as the 'difference principle', although many people now refer to it as 'maximin'. Maximin is a lexicographic principle in that alternative arrangements are compared first from the interests of the least advantaged only. If they are equally badly off under these arrangements, then attention switches to the second least advantaged, and so on.

Rawls defined individual well-being in terms of an index of *primary goods* consisting of: i) basic liberties such as freedom of thought, ii) freedom of choice of occupation, iii) powers and prerogatives of office, iv) income and wealth, and v) social bases of self-respect. This is a rather heterogeneous list and, although Rawls saw income and wealth as acting as more easily measurable proxies for some of the other primary goods, many have criticized him for having a rather vague distribuendum. Moreover, Rawls says very little about how items in the index are to be weighted and so he offers little guidance about how the primary goods are to be traded off against one another in the construction of the index.

However, Rawls does avoid some of the interpersonal comparability problems by defining an 'objective list' of primary goods. This objective list is something which society defines as being important to its *citizens*, as opposed to a welfare economic approach to subjectively valued goods within *consumers'* utility functions. Primary goods would then represent a *subset* of all possible attributes within a consumer's utility function.

Interestingly, Rawls's theory applies only to individuals who are 'normal, active, and fully cooperating members of society over the course of a complete life' (Rawls, 1982). In particular, as noted by Norman Daniels, '*there is no distributive theory for health care because no one is sick*' (Daniels, 1985; italics in original). While the need for Rawls's primary goods, e.g. food and clothing, are more or less the same for all, there is a much more unequal distribution of the need for health care and education, reflecting the 'natural lottery'. There are consequently much wider variations in the resources required to meet such unequal distribution of needs. Applying the maximin principle to health would therefore be a commitment to 'the futile goal of eliminating or "levelling" all natural differences between persons' (Daniels, 1985).

Since the maximin principle owes much to the work of Rawls, it is concerned with the distribution of primary goods, rather than utility or health. However, as with sum ranking, it is entirely reasonable to consider the implications of maximin for any given distribuendum. For example, if the concern were with the distribution of health, then resources would be allocated so as to maximize the health of the most severely ill person. The maximin principle would therefore mean that an individual's *need* for health care is defined according to their *severity of illness*. The lexicographic nature of this principle means that resources would be devoted to the most severely ill individual, or the one with the shortest expected remaining life. Although this decision rule would only apply so long as the expected benefit to the worst-off individual is positive, it would apply irrespective of the benefits forgone by others, even the next-worst-off individual.

An essential aspect of Rawls's theory is to detach people from their own self-interest by concealing their precise position in society. The idea of an *original position* is based upon a view of *justice as impartiality* that argues that an acceptable view for society should reflect agreement between the members of that society. In order to ensure that people's moral decisions are impartial and free from considerations about their own self-interest, people choose the principles of justice for their society from behind a '*veil of ignorance*'. This methodology for choosing between different distributions is referred to as *contractarianism* since each individual from behind the veil agrees to sign up to a social contract, and then the veil is lifted. Rawls held that behind this veil of ignorance individuals will unanimously choose to maximize the primary goods for the worst off, the reason being that each individual will fear being the one who ends up in this position.

The intuitive problem with the maximin solution is its disregard of the forgone utility gains to the better-off group from a marginal improvement for the worst off. Is this a necessary consequence of the just procedure behind the veil of ignorance? Yes, according to Rawlsians; no, according to utilitarians. Both agree on the importance of this 'original position'; that individuals must abstract from selfish interests when judging what is the most just distribution. Harsanyi (1975) holds that 'impartial observers' in their original positions would choose the utilitarian optimum: every individual has an 'equi-probability' of ending up in the different roles. When maximizing their expected utility, individuals will unanimously choose the point in which the average utility is highest, i.e. procedural justice leads to the utilitarian point.

The heart of the disagreement appears to be whether individuals behind the veil of ignorance concentrate their attention upon a non-probabilistic uncertainty, or fear, of ending up as the worst off, or whether they behave as strategic actors who attach probability numbers to the different future roles.

Which distribution of health is fairest?

The differences between the three theories of justice in the context of life-time health can be illustrated by a numerical example. Imagine three countries U(tilia), E(galia) and R(awlia), in each of which there are two groups of people whose respective healthy life expectancies are given in the first row of Table 4.1. Which country is considered to have the fairest distribution of health across the two groups depends on which question on fairness is asked.

Table 4.1 Which distribution of health is fairest?

Healthy life expectancies	U 69 and 78	E 70 and 70	R 71 and 74
Where is the average healthy life expectancy highest?	**73.5**	70	72.5
Where is the distribution of health most equal?	69/78 = 0.88	**70/70 = 1**	71/74 = 0.96
Where is the health of the worst off best?	69	70	**71**

The figures in bold show that utilitarians would opt for U, because this is where the total health is highest; egalitarians would opt for E, because it has the most equal distribution of health; whilst Rawlsians would opt for R, because it is best for the worst off.

4.4 The health frontier and trade-offs

The above theories of justice have been more formally analysed within the framework of the health frontier, in that their respective prescribed solutions are identified as points on the frontier. Trade-offs between these theories can be analysed in terms of social welfare functions.

4.4.1 The health frontier

There are three key assumptions in the health frontier approach:

1. A fixed total health care budget is to be distributed between two (groups of) patients, A and B.

2. The productivity of health care on health is *positive* and the marginal productivity is *diminishing*.

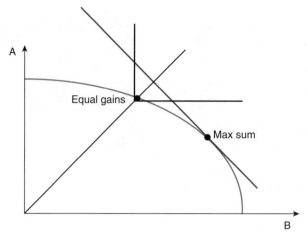

Fig. 4.1 Equality vs efficiency.

3. The health outcomes are measurable on a cardinal scale (e.g. QALYs), and
    are interpersonally comparable.

If the health production functions were similar, the frontier would be symmetric around the 45° equality line from the origin, and hence the health-maximizing allocation would be identical with the egalitarian, as well as the maximin,
solutions. However, the purpose of this frontier is to illustrate the different solutions that emerge when the production functions differ, i.e. when the two (groups
of) patients have different capacities to benefit from health care (see Figure 4.1).
If health maximization were the only policy objective, then this point becomes
the efficient allocation, against which equality is compared.

The shape of the frontier is concave, and hence includes Pareto-efficient
distributions only, i.e. improving the health of one group would imply a reduction in the other group's health. While this shape is something that has very
strong appeal to economists, it reflects a rather restrictive setting. First, it
assumes a fixed health care budget available like 'manna from heaven', something that is relevant in the context of a national health service receiving its
budget like manna from the treasury, and in which people's right to a slice of
the budget is *independent* of their contribution to it. Second, the size of the
budget is independent of how it is distributed between the groups, i.e. there are
no production gains from any of the patient groups that would be channelled
back to the health service in terms of increased tax revenues as a consequence
of having received health care. An inbuilt restriction in this health frontier is
that maximin and equality yield the same solution. In order to have a frontier

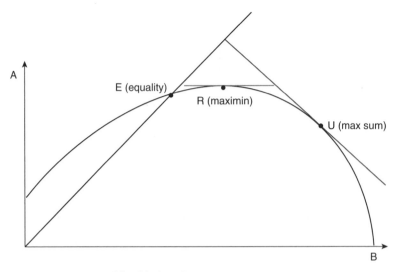

Fig. 4.2 A more general health frontier.

that distinguishes the maximin from the egalitarian point, the frontier would have to include an increasing part. For that to happen, at least one of the above assumptions has to be relaxed.

An explanation for the upward-sloping section from the vertical axis to point R would be that the treatment of A enables him to increase production, which would mean that some of his output could be deployed to the provision of more health care, thereby benefiting the less productive B. In other words, the upward-sloping section illustrates negative net health care costs of treating A, i.e. A would more than 'pay his way' in terms of health care.[3] In Figure 4.2, the total health care budget will increase up to point R.

Figure 4.2 illustrates a more general health frontier that will distinguish the three theories of justice with each respective unique distribution: E involves equal health for A and B, R is the maximin, and U is the maximum total health. Most economists would more or less instinctively focus on the Pareto section, R–U. And, according to Elster (1992), it is between these points that we find distributions that appeal to 'the common-sense conception of justice'. However, if equality per se is part of the health policy objectives, the section E–R may also

---

[3] For an elaboration of this argument, see the model presented in Olsen and Richardson (1999).

become relevant. Points *outside* E–U would not be consistent with any of the above theories of justice.[4]

4.4.2 The social welfare function for health

If people consider both the size of the gains *and* their distribution, the relative weight that they give to these twin considerations will depend on the extent of their equality—efficiency trade-off; that is, the extent to which they prefer equal shares to a greater overall gain. One way to determine this trade-off is to specify a social welfare function (SWF), which would usually include the level of utility of each of two individuals. In this case we consider the health of two individuals, and thus refer to it as a health-related SWF (HRSWF). Most specifications of the SWF assume a constant elasticity of substitution, which means that the curvature of the iso-welfare curve is constant:

$$W = \left[\alpha H_a^{-r} + (1-\alpha)H_b^{-r}\right]^{-\frac{1}{r}}, H_a, H_b \geq 0, \ r \geq -1, \ r \neq 0, \tag{4.2}$$

where:

W = the level of overall population health-related social welfare;

H_a and H_b = the levels of health of A and B;

α = the weight given to one individual relative to the other, as reflected in the *steepness* of the iso-welfare curves;

r = a parameter that measures the degree of aversion to inequality between A and B, as represented by the *convexity* of the iso-welfare curves.

If both individuals are considered to have equal weight, then $\alpha = \frac{1}{2}$, thus resulting in contours that are symmetric around the 45° line. This would be the case when neither of them has any distinguishing extraneous characteristics that would justify treating them differently.

The parameter r measures the strength of equity preferences, i.e. how close to the equity point R the preferred location lies. If $r = -1$, social welfare is equal to the sum of individual utility and thus there is *no* aversion to inequality. This utilitarian-type SWF results in iso-welfare curves that are parallel straight lines with a gradient of $-\alpha/(1-\alpha)$. When $\alpha = \frac{1}{2}$, this gradient is -1. In Equation 4.2, when the two individuals have equal weight, it follows that social welfare is maximized simply by summing their individual health. If $r > -1$, then there is aversion to inequality, i.e. the greater the inequalities between A and B, the

----

[4] For an even more generalized health frontier with a backward-bending part that illustrates the elitist point of maximax, see Olsen (1997).

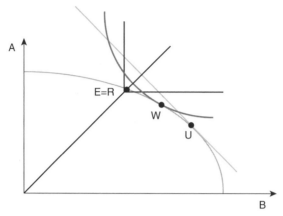

Fig. 4.3 Trade-offs: maximum HRSW.

greater the weight given to the worst-off individual relative to the better-off one. This results in iso-welfare curves that are *convex* to the origin. In the extreme, the worst-off individual is all that matters and r takes a value of infinity. This will result in a Rawlsian-type SWF with L-shaped (or right-angled) iso-welfare curves. Thus, the higher the parameter value of r, the stronger the equity preferences, i.e. the closer one gets to the equity point, which is also the Rawlsian point R, and hence further away from the utilitarian point U. Figure 4.3 shows these various SWFs (all with $\alpha = \frac{1}{2}$).

This discussion of distributive justice has located three analytically different points on the health possibility frontier (HPF), all of which are equally good according to the Pareto criterion. These points are: U, the sum-ranking solution suggested by utilitarians; R, the maximin solution associated with Rawls; and W, a trade-off solution following from a SWF which makes trade-offs between the arguments of the former two (corner) solutions. The actual location of this third point critically depends on the degree of aversion to inequality.

The point at which the iso-welfare curve is tangential to the health frontier represents the optimal distribution of health gains across the two patients. In the jargon of microeconomics, at this point the marginal rate of substitution equals the marginal rate of transformation, which again reflects the opportunity costs of equity in terms of health benefits forgone for B for an additional unit of health gain for A. Hence, the more equality-prone you are, the higher the opportunity cost of equity.

Most of the literature on the health frontier and the HRSWF has considered one 'stream of health' only, namely prospective gains. It is implicitly, and sometimes explicitly, assumed that all other streams of health are identical, such as the individual's age and the health remaining to them without treatment. Chapter 15 will explore this issue of 'equality of what' in more detail.

The opportunity cost (= benefits forgone) of equity

Imagine a given health care budget that can produce different amounts of health to A and B depending on how we split the budget between the two. At one extreme everything is spent on A (A_{max}), at the other extreme everything is spent on B (B_{max}). In allocation II the budget is split so that A and B receive the same gains (6 each), while allocations V and VI both involve maximum total health (18). The last column shows the opportunity costs in terms of benefits forgone to B for each additional unit of health gained for A.

Table 4.2 The opportunity cost (= benefits forgone) of equity

	A	B	Sum total	Benefits forgone to B for 1 more to A
I A_{max}	7	0	7	−6
II Equality	6	6	12	−4
III	5	10	15	−3
IV	4	13	17	−2
V Max sum	3	15	18	−1
VI Max sum	2	16	18	−0.7
VII	1	16.7	17.7	−0.3
VIII B_{max}	0	17	17	

Which allocation would you prefer? If you are an egalitarian (or Rawlsian) you would opt for II; if you are a health-maximizing utilitarian, you would opt for V (or VI); or you might wish to make a trade-off between the two corner principles. In so doing you might take a look at the final column and be confronted with 'the price of equity'.

4.5 Conclusion and some conceptual clarifications

The 'ethics of economics' owe much to the utilitarian philosophy. When economists are accused of being preoccupied with efficiency and maximization issues, they can at least justify this obsession by reference to an important philosophical school of thought. There are two different sets of arguments against this utilitarian concept of justice and fairness. The first argues in favour of alternative points *on* the utility possibility frontier to the utilitarian sum-ranking point. The suggested alternative points would reflect some notions of equity. These could be based on a Rawlsian argument of maximizing the utility of the worst off, a preference for equal distribution of goods, or preferences for an intermediate point on the frontier that would balance the twin aims of maximizing the total sum of utilities and of having an equal distribution. Still, while disagreeing with the utilitarian solution, these alternatives have a consequentialistic focus.

The second set of arguments against utilitarianism shares a basis in procedural justice. Important here are various notions of citizens' rights. People appear to have a wide range of concepts of what is involved in considering human beings as being equally entitled to—and worthy of—care. Furthermore, most of us would require legal justice and democratic principles to be followed. Interestingly, it might well be an implication of a procedural justice argument to opt for a point *inside* the health frontier. It is indeed a challenge to try and distinguish those inefficient distributions that have an explanation in procedural justice and fairness from those which represent mere waste—and a further challenge to consider whether the price (in terms of forgone benefits) of fair procedures is a price worth paying or not.

In this chapter we have—consistent with the wider literature on equality and fairness in health and health care—come to apply some overlapping concepts such as equity and justice. Some conceptual clarification might therefore be helpful.

4.5.1 **Equality**

Equality means equal division of the distribuendum (the entity to be distributed) or equalisandum (the entity of which we want an equal distribution). Admittedly, different authors have not always been precise regarding what the entity is. It might be income, wealth, utility, well-being, primary goods, opportunities, circumstances, basic capabilities, or—in the current context—health or health care. Some of these entities are hard to measure, and some of them have an instrumental purpose in that they are believed to be important for the good we are seeking, which most likely is some sort of well-being.

Good health makes people capable of flourishing in other important walks of life (Culyer, 1989). There are positive side effects from improved health in terms of wealth (through labour force participation) and social relations, including wider participation in communal life. Hence, aiming for *equality in health* seems partly to be motivated by aiming for equal opportunities to flourish.

Equality of health care is normally put with the added 'equal access (to health care) for equal need'. Note the two provisos: i) *access*, as opposed to utilization, means that inequalities in health care use due to variations in preferences would normally be acceptable, and ii) *equal need* means that health care should *not* be distributed independently of variations in needs, i.e. 'unequals should be treated unequally'. The concept of *need* therefore becomes crucial in health economics.

In everyday language, *need* is often taken to express the degree of urgency for health care, i.e. 'need as ill health' in terms of the expected no-treatment profile or severity of a patient's illness. Among most health economists, need is a concept that refers to the degree of potential benefits from treatment, i.e. 'need as capacity to benefit'. Hence, in order to comply with both of these contrasting interpretations, the slogan 'equal access for equal need' must mean equal capacity to benefit from an equal initial state of ill health.

4.5.2 **Equity = equal shares or justifiably unequal shares**

A leading health economist in this field, Tony Culyer, holds that: 'Plainly, there is no single, universal theory of equity, but it is widely agreed that *equity* implies *equality*. Unfortunately, there is no accord concerning *what* should be equal' (2001; italics in original). Clearly, the reverse does not hold. If it did, the concepts of equality and equity would be synonymous.

As to the issue of *what* should be equal, the health economics literature has been concerned with equal choices and equal opportunities. Two decades ago, Le Grand (1987) argued that inequalities in health care use are not inequitable if they result from different choices or preferences. Hence, according to this line of reasoning it follows that those inequalities in health that emerge from an equal 'choice set' are considered equitable.

Horizontal equity requires the like treatment of like individuals, and vertical equity requires the unlike treatment of *unlike* individuals. The crucial issue then is to identify the morally relevant characteristics that would justify that individuals become 'unlike' in terms of their entitlements to health care.

While the concept of equity is closely intertwined with equality, so it is with fairness. In *Handbook of Health Economics*, Alan Williams and Richard Cookson hold that: 'In economics the term "equity" is usually taken to refer to fairness in the distribution of a good (in this case "health"), and "fairness" is taken almost unthinkingly to mean reducing inequalities' (Williams and Cookson, 2000). With this in mind, as well as Culyer's view on equity vs equality, it is tempting to suggest that *equity implies equality and/or fair inequalities*.

4.5.3 **Fairness: some diverse interpretations**

Fairness is a word with seemingly only positive connotations. It refers to what is intuitively right, acceptable or just. Within health economics the concept of fairness has primarily been used in relation to equity.

However, a completely contrasting perception of fairness in the health economics literature is the concept of 'actuarial fairness', something which will be discussed in Chapter 7 on health insurance. Strongly related to this idea of fairness is that of what is deserved in terms of a link between effort and reward. It is one thing to divide 'manna from heaven'; it is another to divide a pie the size of which depends on differences in contributions and efforts among those who will eat it.

Another concept of fairness in the economics literature is that of 'fairness as non-envy': when no agent wishes to hold any other agent's final bundle, this is an equitable allocation (Varian, 1975). Note that the distribuendum is no longer uni-dimensional (e.g. income), but multiple (e.g. leisure and income). Applied in a health economics context this could be presented as a choice between bundles of health and wealth: A (80 QALYs, €60,000 annual income) and B (70 QALYs, €80,000 annual income). If Ann prefers A and Betty prefers B, then it is fair—simply because they would not swap.[5] However, this concept of fairness as non-envy has received little attention in the health economics literature, in which much of the concern for equity and fairness has dealt with partial distributions of a uni-dimensional good, such as number of QALYs.

4.5.4 Justice = just procedures + just distributions

While the concept of fairness may give a broad set of connotations reflecting the many situations in everyday life for which it is being used, the concept of justice is somewhat more 'professional' and often associated with the disciplines of philosophy, law, and political science. When health economists have applied theories of justice, they have primarily dealt with those theories of distributive justice that can ascribe solutions identified as points on a health possibility frontier. Elster (1992) makes an interesting observation when suggesting that 'the task of the major theories of justice can be stated as *justifying deviations from equality* ... the burden of proof is on the advocate of an unequal distribution' (italics in original). In the context of Figure 4.2, Rawlsians would justify a move from E to R, because it benefits the worst off. Utilitarians would justify a further movement from R to U by reference to 'the greatest happiness principle': as long as the loss to the worst off is less than the gain to the better off, the sum total increases.

Furthermore, if concerned with providing equal 'choice sets'—or *equal opportunities*—an unequal distribution may be justified on the grounds that it

---

[5] In practice health and wealth are not inversely correlated as the examples may suggest. Generally, the healthy are also the wealthy.

results from well-informed choices among individuals who have faced equal opportunities. And if you take an admittedly extreme libertarian view, whatever distribution emerges may be justified as long as it results from just procedures regarding respect for liberties and duties.

Suggested reading

Daniels, N. (2008) *Just Health: Meeting Health Needs Fairly*. New York: Cambridge University Press.

Roemer, J. (1996) *Theories of Distributive Justice*. Harvard University Press.

Culyer, A. J. (2007) Equity of what in health care? Why the traditional answers don't help policy—and what to do in the future. *Healthcare Papers*, 8 (Sp), 12–26.

McInture, D. and Mooney, G. (eds) (2007) The economics of health equity, Cambridge University Press, Cambridge.

Exercises

1. Why do we care for other people's access to health care?

2. Discuss the concept of 'need' for health care: 'need as ill health' vs 'need as capacity to benefit'.

3. Think of some real world resource allocation cases in health care justified on procedural justice that clearly have led to some inefficient outcomes. Explain.

Part 2

Intervening in the determinants of health

The crucial public health question, 'Why are some people healthy and others not?' is discussed in a book with the same title by Evans *et al.* (1994). They consider there to be three major determinants of (ill) health in a population. First, *genetics*, which explains inherited diseases through natural variations in human biology. Second, *the environment*, including such physical factors as working conditions and pollution, and social factors such as cultural norms and position in the social hierarchy. And third, (health-related) *lifestyle*, which at the population level can be explained largely by cultural and social norms.

The three determinants differ in the extent to which individuals can exercise discretion and control over them. Genetic endowments are something that most of us take as given, no matter how hard we might fight against them. The physical and social environment represents the circumstances under which people live. These circumstances are to a large extent given, particularly for children, who have very little say over the environment they are brought up in. If they were to have a say, we might have very different social arrangements and very different views about what constitutes social injustice. As we get older, we come to have more freedom in choosing the environment but we are never completely without constraints.

Lifestyle is the determinant of ill health over which we have most discretion, but precisely how much of observed behaviour reflects genuine choice and how much is due to factors outside the individual's control is a very contentious issue. Rather than consider lifestyle to be entirely within an individual's control or to be entirely determined by genetic and environmental factors, it is more helpful to consider an individual's lifestyle to be determined by a variety of factors over which they have differing *degrees of discretion*.

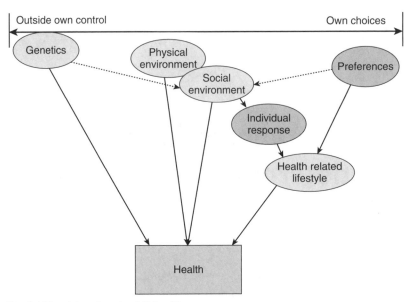

Fig. 5.1 The determinants of ill health.

Figure 5.1 gives a graphical representation of the determinants of ill health. We have chosen to introduce *preferences* (rather than lifestyle) as an independent variable. This variable is to reflect genuine differences in the choices that people make. Note here that a particular preference is not unhealthy per se. It is when a preference is being *revealed through behaviour* that it may become unhealthy. An individual's lifestyle, then, depends upon a combination of their *responses* to the environment and their *choices* determined by their freely expressed preferences. In reality, of course, genetics, environment, and preferences are related to one another, but for ease of exposition all of the possible arrows between them are not shown here. Among these determinants, the first two—at least in principle—are observable, whilst preferences are not. Health-related lifestyle, however, is observable.

The emphasis on health-related lifestyle within this map of causation is justified on the grounds that this variable is often associated with self-inflicted diseases, for which, some would argue, individuals should be held *responsible*. However, the model suggests that a 'lifestyle disease' is not necessarily self-inflicted; rather it may be caused by a mental or biological response to the environment in which a person happens to find themselves.

The map of causality in Figure 5.1 illustrates the determinants at which various public health interventions could be targeted. Genetics will not be discussed any further, as it is a determinant that we cannot influence (at least not in the short run).

Chapter 5

The health environment

This chapter discusses some key policy options for reducing the negative impacts of an unhealthy environment, as well as some challenges involved when attempting to reduce social causes of ill health.

By definition, an unhealthy environment creates ill health, and thereafter more need for health care. Studying the various impacts from the environment on human health, through human biology pathways, lies outside the field of economics. The focus here will be on some economic principles for interventions, for the purpose of reducing the negative environmental impacts on health.

5.1 The physical environment

In the current context, we are interested in the physical environment to the extent that it has negative health impacts, through human biology pathway or stress censors. Air pollution beyond a certain level may create respiratory diseases. Polluted water and pesticides contaminate the water we drink and the food we eat, something which will affect the digestive system. Nuclear waste will through radiation increase the risks of cancer and of having deformed children. And finally, noise may reduce hearing and/or create stress.

The economic problem with an unhealthy physical environment is that it represents a 'public bad' in terms of health to individuals. As explained in Chapter 3 on market failures, a *public good* is characterized by non-rivalry (many consumers can benefit simultaneously without reducing each individual's own benefit) and non-excludability (people can receive benefits without having paid). With a public bad all individuals are harmed simultaneously, and there is no incentive for one individual to pay to reduce the problem.

In the same way as an unregulated market will *under*-provide public goods, so will an unregulated market *over*-provide public bads. The classic example of a public bad is that of pollution.

The *territory* of a public bad may vary considerably, anything from the problem of global warming through to a polluted city or down to bad smell in a shared office. The choice for the individual being affected is basically one of 'Should I stay or should I go?'. While you could leave the office, and move from a polluted city, it is more difficult to move from the earth! No wonder, therefore, about global concern about climate change.

There are two sets of challenges regarding interventions: i) how to raise the funding for cleaning up an unhealthy physical environment, and ii) how to make those who produce public bads stop doing so.

As to fund raising, tax financing is the standard solution. However, rather than this type of coerced contribution, there are variants in terms of voluntary contributions, e.g. CO_2 certificates when purchasing airline tickets. Nonetheless, it makes more sense to reduce the production of public bads in the first place. In general, economists have a strong affinity to the polluter pay principle (PPP) rather than direct regulations through jurisdiction. The underlying idea behind PPP is very simple: in addition to the internal production costs faced by the firm, the negative externality imposed on others as part of the production process involves a disutility that can be measured as an additional cost that the decision maker should be confronted with, i.e. 'externalities should be internalized'. Or, to put it simply and formally: private marginal costs (PC) + external costs (EC) = social marginal costs (SC).

Figure 5.2 shows the market demand curve or the social benefits (SB), the private supply curve that reflects the marginal costs to the firm for each unit

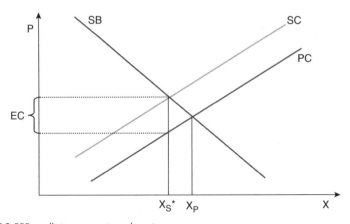

Fig. 5.2 PPP: polluter pay external costs.

produced (*PC*), and the social cost curve (*SC*). The vertical distance between the two cost curves illustrates the magnitude of the negative externalities imposed on others (*EC*). The socially optimal quantity, X_S^*, is determined where the social marginal costs equal the social marginal benefits, i.e. the intersection between *SC* and *SB*.

In terms of environmental policies, there are many real world examples of how indirect taxation is levied on negative externalities. Congestion charges for driving private vehicles into central London is one such.

In Figure 5.2 the distance between the two cost curves (*SC—PC*) indicates a fixed increase in external costs (health damages caused by increasing emissions) with increasing production. However, in the same way as the carrying capacity of the ecological system might hit a threshold beyond which nature cannot absorb more emissions, the same might happen with the health damage caused by emissions: beyond a given level, human biology cannot absorb more.

Figure 5.3 illustrates such a case. The initial quantity X_P is determined by the intersection between the private cost curve, *PC*, and the demand curve, *SB*. Negative health effects are identified and it is decided to reduce the quantity to a socially optimal level: X_S. The policy solution is one of PPP, i.e. introduce an indirect tax that reflect the external costs, t_E. The consequence of this is that X_S is determined in the intersection between the social cost curve ($SC = PC + t_E$) and the demand curve.

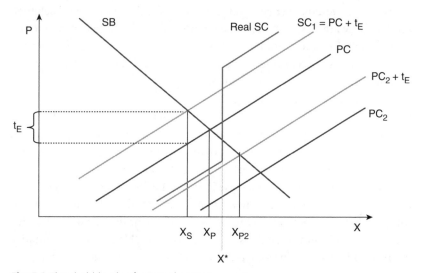

Fig. 5.3 Threshold levels of external costs.

What happens if a technology improvement in private production yields lower private costs, illustrated by a shift in the private cost curve from PC to PC_2? Then, with the current indirect tax, the producer is faced with the cost curve $(PC_2 + t_E)$, that intersects the demand curve at a higher quantity, X_{P2}, than the initial X_P. The problem now is that X_{P2} involves a production level that has created emissions beyond a threshold level X^*, at which there is a dramatic increase in health damage. Hence, in situations where increased emissions may reach a threshold level beyond which health damage becomes severe, the policy implications would be to opt for emission quotas or other types of direct regulation. (A textbook on environmental economics will provide more background on the pros and cons of direct and indirect regulation of pollution.)

In the current context of health damage, externalities can be identified on two fronts. First, internally in the production process when workers' health is being negatively affected, in terms of either a more permanent health deterioration or an increased risk of accidents. The economic problem is that employers do not pay the full costs of labour as an input factor, which in Marxist terminology would be considered a type of *exploitation*. The way to internalize such externalities would be introduce safety legislation that forces employers to improve the work environment and implement safety measures. Alternatively, employers would have to make financial compensation to those workers who are prepared to make trade-offs between health risks and earnings.

The other type of health externality is apparent literally outside the factory building, i.e. as emissions in the neighbouring communities. Again, policy interventions would either be direct regulation of emissions to a level below an acceptable health risk, or to have the polluting firm pay sufficient compensation to the affected communities. The optimal level of such compensation would be assessed according to the value of the health consequences or the disutility among the affected individuals.

The types of health damage consequent upon environmental exposure would in most cases be a small degree of damage for many people rather than large losses for a few. Pollution in various forms involves long-term health damage that yields further deterioration in human biology (see Figure 1.1). Interventions that seek to avoid such health damage could be valued in terms of the avoided increase in future health care costs. However, it clearly makes more sense to justify environmental health interventions for their health benefits (= avoided health deterioration) rather than for their expected health service cost savings. As such, this type of preventative interventions should—in principle—be analysed using the same methodologies as any other health intervention (see Part 5 of this book).

5.2 **The social environment**

There is now increasing evidence of a strong correlation between social position and health. This 'social gradient' has been identified using various indicators, such as income, education level, social class, as well as people's position in
a social hierarchy. The higher up the social ladder, the better the individual's
health. This holds not only for human beings but has been documented in
other species as well.

The observed social inequalities in health have received much attention in
many countries. Policy makers with an egalitarian affinity consider such
inequalities to be unfair, because they are *avoidable*—if only society had done
something about it. The challenge is to find effective interventions that will
reduce these inequalities.

However, before choosing an intervention, one would need to establish that
the observed positive *correlation* represents a *causality*, i.e. social class $\uparrow \rightarrow$
health$\uparrow$. If education level is used as an indicator for social class, and a positive
correlation is observed between education and health, the policy prescription
would be to increase the level of education at the bottom end. The hypothe-
sized causality is that more education makes people better informed to make
healthy choices.

Clearly, at low absolute income levels people become deprived from living a
healthy life when they cannot afford food, shelter and medical treatments.
Income support for such groups would then be a sensible intervention for
improving their health, and hence reducing social inequalities in health. Things
become more complicated when analysing population groups with absolute
income levels significantly above subsistence level. At such income levels, it is
not the *absolute* income that restricts people from living a healthy life. Rather,
it may be the *relative* income inequalities that matter.

Comparisons between countries suggest that life expectancies are higher
in countries with more equal distribution of income. In general, the more
unequal the income distribution, the more people will consider it unfair. An
unequal income distribution is a public bad in that it creates a social environment of distrust, lack of respect, and aggression—factors that affect the health
of all members of society.[1] Conversely, a fair income distribution would be
considered a public good that—for reasons of trust, respect, and a calmer
social climate—would be health enhancing to everybody. Hence, the intervention becomes one of income redistribution.

---

[1] See Wilkinson, R. G. (1996) *Unhealthy societies: the affliction of inequality*, London,
Routledge.

Beyond being a public good (or public bad), an individual's own place in the income distribution is a private good (or bad) that signals social position. When the individual is using their own income for assessing their positional value, the question is: who is the reference group? Does the individual compare their income with the average of their cohort, their class from college, or their colleagues? If income plays a role in signalling social position, and social position is what matters to people's health, then the individual's *ordinal* place in the income distribution would matter more than the magnitude of the inequalities per se. So while a policy intervention of progressive taxation will reduce income inequalities, it does not necessarily reduce health inequalities—if the underlying mechanism is a link between social hierarchy and health.

Interestingly, the reference group becomes wider when social mobility is high (i.e. equal opportunities to climb up the social ladder, and high risk of falling down). The individual's success or failure at work would then to a large extent depend on their own efforts and abilities. If on the other hand social mobility is low, they could blame external societal mechanisms for not having provided them with the opportunities to succeed. Hence, when a country increases its social mobility, each individual's reference group becomes wider. The relative deprivation increases among those who have not succeeded, something that has negative health effects. Say an individual has an income of 20 and the income span in society ranges from 10 to 100. If their reference group were narrow, say between 10 and 30, the individual would not consider themselves a social failure. Given the links between *relative* social position and health (see below) this issue of a widening social reference group may be one reason why social inequalities in health have persisted despite the many health policy measures that have improved access to health irrespective of income.[2]

The correlation between income and health is measurable and indisputable: the wealthy are also the healthy. However, the degree of causality is certainly more controversial (remember, the healthy are also the wealthy!). While the goodness and badness of a certain income distribution is a heated political issue, the controversy in the scientific community deals with the difficulties in tracing the complete pathway that goes from relative income to health. Recent attempts at explaining this pathway seem to emphasize the importance of social position. Relative income is important as a signal of relative social position, and social position gives social status. Income then becomes a 'conspicuous good' to signal social status.

---

[2] While this mechanism is a negative side effect of increased social mobility, one may still be a passionate supporter of the principle of equal opportunities.

Rather than using relative income as an indicator for social position, we could study the association between social class and health, as well as the association between people's position in a social hierarchy and their health. The UK system of six 'social classes' is categorized by occupations only. Recent data shows that British males in the professional class have a life expectancy of 80 years, compared with 72.7 for those in the manual unskilled class. Although life expectancies have increased in all social classes over the last 30-year period, the *relative* difference in life expectancy between the manual unskilled compared with the professional class has persisted.[3] Interestingly, the social class variation in health is stronger among males than females, something which suggests that men are more sensitive to social position, or that men's identity at work is more important to their overall well-being.

One of the most cited studies on the association between the individual's position in an organizational hierarchy and health is the British study of government employees (commonly referred to as the Whitehall study).[4]

The explanation for the worse health at the bottom of social hierarchies is that people with low social status have weaker social relationships, they get less approval and support, and they have less self-control. This social-psychological pathway is associated with stress. In neuroscience the term 'allostatic load' is used as a measure of cumulative stress. It is a composite index of indicators of cumulative strain on multiple organs and tissues, which accumulates via the wear and tear associated with acute shifts in physiologic activity in response to negative stimuli.[5] Differences in allostatic load may reflect differences in stress exposure. In the same way as there exist threshold levels for pollution beyond which an ecosystem cannot self-clean, the level of cumulative stress may reach thresholds beyond which the human organism cannot cope. The immune system is then affected, and people become more susceptible to various diseases. Hence, *a social-psychological pathway is followed by biological pathways.*

Interventions to reduce social inequalities in health are often controversial, as they have societal implications far beyond health policy. Redistributing income

---

[3] In the period 1972—75, life expectancy of a manual unskilled male was 92.5% of that of a male from the professional class (66.5 years / 71.9 years). In the period 2002–05 the relative difference had increased slightly to 91% (72.7 years / 80 years) http://www.statistics. gov.uk/pdfdir/le1007.pdf

[4] Marmot, M. (2004) *The status syndrome: How social standing affects our health and longevity*, Times Books, New York.

[5] http://en.wikipedia.org/wiki/Allostatic_load

and wealth might well reduce health inequalities, and possibly improve health for all groups in society, but might still be impossible to implement for other reasons, e.g. it might be considered unfair to tax people more heavily. Interventions targeted at empowering people at the lower end of social hierarchies might be opposed by those who hold power at the top. Clearly, there must be a range of workplace intervention that will reduce social position-type stress, but that lies outside the scope of this book.

Nevertheless, no matter how strong any public health interventions that are implemented, some social inequalities in health are unavoidable. This is due to the existence of underlying variables that have an impact in the same direction on both variables under study, i.e. factors that determine social position as well as health. First, natural variations from birth imply that our biological preconditions for social success (shown in Figure 5.1 as the dotted arrow from genetics to social environment), as well as good health later in life, will differ. Interventions such as maternity care and early childhood follow up will help reduce the influence of this determinant of social inequalities in health, i.e. inequalities that are being reproduced through generations.

Second, people have different personality traits: ambitious people with low time preferences and much self-control will put more effort into their social standing as well as their health. To the extent that people choose their social class, they may end up where health-related habits and culture best correspond with their personality traits (shown in Figure 5.1 as the dotted arrow from preferences to social environment). Later adaption to social norms, or social conditioning, will thereby reinforce health-related choices.

5.3 Conclusion

The physical and social environments discussed here represent the *circumstances* under which people live and to which they more or less have to adapt. While there are certainly links between these two sets of determinants (physical environment influences social environment, and vice versa), this issue lies outside the scope of this book. The important distinction to be made here is that physical and social environments represent more structural constraints, while health-related lifestyle to a larger extent reflects *choices* based on individual preferences.

Suggested reading

Evans, R. G., Barer, M. L. and Marmor, T. R. (ed.) (1994) *Why are some people healthy and others not? The determinants of health of populations.* New York: Aldine de Gruyter.

Hanley, N., Shogren, J. F. and White, B. (2001) *Introduction to Environmental Economics.* Oxford: Oxford University Press.

Marmot, M. (2004) *The status syndrome: How social standing affects our health and longevity.* New York: Times Books.

Marmot, M. (2007) Achieving health equity: from root causes to fair outcomes. *Lancet*, 370, 1153–63.

Exercises

1. Consider an environmental health issue in your community or town, and discuss which interventions are possible to reduce its negative health impacts.

2. Explore available official statistics in your country that may indicate the extent of social inequalities in health. Can you observe social inequalities in *children's* health?

3. To what extent do you think there is a positive association between a healthy *physical* environment and a healthy *social* environment? Find examples and evidence.

Chapter 6

Health-related lifestyle

This chapter explores alternative interventions in people's health-related behaviour, for the purpose of making us choose a healthy diet, exercise more, and reduce the use of substances. Various direct regulations are discussed, as well as indirect regulations through the price mechanism.

Imagine a health-neutral behaviour that yields a 'health span' as illustrated in Figure 1.1. The health-related lifestyle that we observe in people would to various extents be either healthy in terms of enhancing this health span or unhealthy in terms of something that would deteriorate this health span. When we talk about healthy or unhealthy lifestyle, we are referring to the observed choices people make regarding their diet, their exercise, and their substance use.

Although life expectancies are increasing in most countries, there is much concern that large fractions of the population have an unhealthy lifestyle: First, there is an 'obesity epidemic' in rich countries. Two-thirds of the US adult population is now classified as overweight (body mass index (BMI) > 25).[1] Half of them—one third of the population—are obese (BMI > 30). The increased BMI is caused essentially by changes in diet and exercise, i.e. more sugar and fat food combined with less physical activity. While this change in behaviour can be interpreted as a 'rational response' to increased wealth, its consequences are still deteriorated health.

Second, substance use (and abuse) is changing. Rich countries are using less tobacco while poor countries are using more. Generally, alcohol consumption

---

[1] BMI is measured as an individual's weight in kilograms (kg) divided by height in metres (m) squared; e.g. weight 72 kg and height 1.80 m gives a BMI of 72/(1.80 x 1.80) = 22.2.

increases with wealth. While some use of alcohol might be healthy in terms of reduced cardiovascular diseases, excessive use is certainly unhealthy. Illegal substances are in general unhealthy, but the use of some types of narcotics is still increasing.

A recurrent policy issue is how far the 'nanny state' should interfere in individuals' health-related choices. What is the problem with an unhealthy lifestyle and for *whom* is it a problem? One problem is that an unhealthy lifestyle leads to more need for health care, and hence increased health care costs. However, if the health insurance premiums we pay reflect our expected health care costs, then the cost of an unhealthy lifestyle is something that each individual is being confronted with. Obese smokers would simply have to pay a higher health insurance premium than slim non-smokers. So the associated increased health care costs of an unhealthy lifestyle are in principle not a costing problem in risk-based health insurance (see Chapter 7), simply because the costs are being paid by those who will later come to need health care.

Under social insurance or tax-financed health care there is no link between own premium/contribution and own expected health care costs. In this case the increased health care costs associated with an unhealthy lifestyle are being imposed on those with a healthy lifestyle. While there are strong efficiency and equity reasons for a health care system in which there is no link between our expected health care costs and our financial contribution, an inbuilt feature of this system is the complete lack of financial incentive for choosing the healthy way. Thus, there is a policy challenge to make people face the cost consequences of their health related choices, i.e. make them 'internalize the externalities'.

Beyond health care cost externalities there may be other types of externalities on others—e.g. passive smoking—as well externalities on oneself in the future: addiction and 'weak will' may call for interventions justified on the grounds of what we referred to in Chapter 4 as 'soft paternalism'. Like the interventions discussed in Chapter 5, the health policy options available for altering people's health-related lifestyle are either direct regulations (e.g. smoking laws) or indirect regulations (e.g. tobacco taxes).

6.1 Diet

Diet is probably the most important determinant of health, in terms of both quantity and quality. Clearly, too little or too much intake of food is unhealthy. When it comes to defining best quality in terms of nutritional value, food experts may dispute. But there appears to be a wide level of agreement on the following: fruit, vegetables, fat fish, and olive oil are good for us, while sugar, butter, red meat, and salt are bad for us.

Food is truly a *necessity* in the everyday meaning of the word, but also when used as an economic concept (see Chapter 2). When comparing household spending patterns across income levels, richer households spend relatively less of their income on food than do poorer ones (though of course the rich may still spend more on food in absolute terms). Such comparisons over time show that the proportion of the household budget spent on food is declining, e.g. from around 40% to around 10% in rich countries such as Norway and the UK over the last 50 years. In poor countries the current budget proportion for food is still more than 50% of household income. At the bottom end, the poorest households living at subsistence level might spend all of their income on food.

Despite the fact that people spend a decreasing fraction of their income on food, there is much consumer focus on food prices. In many countries, unhealthy food is relatively cheap, while healthy food is relatively expensive. Therefore, intervening in the relative prices of food seems—at least in theory—a sensible health policy option. The more *unhealthy* a type of food is, the higher it should be *taxed*; and the more *healthy* a type of food is, the better reason to *subsidize* it. The most important issue is the quantity reaction to changing prices, or the elasticity of demand. If the demand for a particular food is inelastic, large relative changes in taxes and subsidies are called for in order to obtain the desired quantity reaction.

Because low-income groups spend a higher share of their budget on food, they are more sensitive to price changes than are rich people. And because poor people spend relatively more of their income on unhealthy food, taxing these goods would then have relatively more negative impact on poor people's incomes. However, the net food-tax burden of this type of food policy does not have to be negative, if the savings from subsidized healthy food outweigh the increased expenditure on unhealthy food.

In general, the lower the share of budget spent on goods whose prices are being changed, the less the reaction, i.e. the more inelastic the demand. For instance, the price of salt would have to increase by an extreme amount to have a deterrent effect on salt intake beyond the recommended level of some few grams per day. In such cases direct regulations, e.g. through information campaigns, might prove to be more effective policy options.

Note that a food policy of interventions in relative prices, though subsidizing healthy food and taxing unhealthy food, does not have to result in a net expense to the treasury: the total public expenditure on subsidies for healthy food do not have to be larger than the total revenues from taxes on unhealthy food. However, if it so happens that the net effect turns out to be negative for the public purse, it might still be a cost-effective health intervention. It depends on the health gains from the changed diet following such a food policy.

6.2 **Exercise**

An increasing number of us spend most of the working day on a chair staring at a computer screen. People in rich countries spend less time being physically active. Hence, when work does not oblige us to be physically active, we may choose to be inactive. The problem is that inactivity is unhealthy, because the human body was designed for some level of activity. Which types of interventions would make people more physically active?

There are two principal types of intervention, taking account of the distinction between choices and circumstances. Circumstances in this context refer to how 'exercise-friendly' people's choice sets happen to be, e.g. the existence cycle paths, running tracks, and swimming pools. Interventions could then be targeted at making those options available to people that require exercise, as well as making lazy options less attractive, e.g. making driving to work more expensive.

Individual choices regarding physical activity can be altered through incentives. Health insurance companies might offer cheaper premiums to customers who join a gym, and employers might allow employees paid time off for exercise. Note that these types of incentives are motivated by the positive externalities that physical activity have on other agents, e.g. in terms of fewer insurance claims and higher productivity. As such, the incentives are *not* motivated by the improved health or the increased energy that yield utility to the individual.

If individuals know that it is in their best interest to exercise, but they lack the will to exercise, there is a case for some 'soft paternalist' interventions. An example would be the introduction of exercise schemes that have inbuilt incentives for pre-commitment, i.e. the individual could choose to sign up to a contract that penalizes the future bad behaviour they currently wish to avoid, while rewarding the future good behaviour they currently aspire to.

6.3 **Substance use**

By substances in this context we refer to tobacco, alcohol, narcotics, and even caffeine, i.e. things we can eat, drink, smoke, or inject that in their different ways are detrimental to human biology—at least when consumed beyond a given quantity.[2] In addition to their detrimental health effects, some substances are very addictive. Note that addiction per se is a separate issue from the health effects of substance use. Hence, intervention for reasons of avoiding *addiction* has a different rationale from that of avoiding *ill health*.

---

[2] It may be more customary to use the terms substance *mis*use or substance *ab*use.

6.3.1 **Tobacco**

Tobacco is one of the most addictive substances available. In fact, most smokers wish they had not started. This in itself should justify interventions that make the substance less available for potentially new users.

There is now plenty of evidence that daily smoking is the major cause of lung cancer, that it increases the risk of other types of cancer, and has many other negative effects on health: every cigarette increases the risk of cancer and deteriorates the respiratory and cardiovascular systems. This ill health leads to increased costs to the health service. However, there is one very simple policy solution to this financial externality: levying a tax on tobacco that goes to financing the increased health care costs. So if smokers 'pay their way' in terms of tobacco taxes—i.e. tobacco tax revenue equals the increased costs of treating diseases attributable to smoking—smokers cannot then be blamed for imposing a cost burden on non-smoking taxpayers.

However, smoking may impose other types of externalities on others. There is some evidence of health damage from passive smoking, at least among those who are exposed to this for long periods, such as employees in bars and restaurants.[3] Beyond ill health, the majority of non-smokers simply dislike being exposed to smoke—just as with any other type of pollution. Hence, the basis for an optimal tobacco tax should in principle include two types of externalities: the financial externality on the health service from treating smoking-related diseases (as well as those that may follow from passive smoking) plus compensation for the disutility experienced among non-smokers.

Since the latter type of compensation is hard to put into practice—e.g. that non-smokers would actually receive a financial compensation for allowing a smoker to light up a cigarette, there is an argument for direct regulation such as banning smoking in public places. This type of intervention aimed at non-smokers' right to clean air has created heated debates in most countries.

6.3.2 **Alcohol**

While tobacco is a substance that has no positive health effects, alcohol consumption up to a certain level may in fact have positive effects on the cardiovascular system. The problem, though, is that increased alcohol intake has increasing detrimental effects on health. But the most severe externality relates to excess alcohol consumption, through social costs imposed on others.

---

[3] In fact, this was one of the key arguments used for banning smoking in bars and restaurants in Norway.

These various effects of alcohol reflect the various levels at which it is consumed. Interestingly, small quantities may be healthy, intermediate quantities may be unhealthy (though many well-informed individuals appreciate the sedative or recreational effects of alcohol), while large quantities ('binge drinking') have inebriant or intoxicant effects. The challenge for policy makers when implementing alcohol interventions is to acknowledge these diverse and contrasting effects of alcohol. At small quantities, the optimal intervention is to subsidize it in accordance with its positive health externalities; at intermediate quantities, it should be taxed on the basis of its health care costs externalities; and at larger quantities, it should be taxed even further to cover the additional social costs, perhaps along with strong direct regulation to restrict its access.

The problem in practice is of course that one cannot implement different price distortions on the same product for different consumption groups. The reason for avoiding extremely high taxes on alcohol, or to restrict its access among problem users, is that alternative illegal access is always an option, e.g. illegal distilling, smuggling, and the possibility that some user groups might switch to illicit drugs.

So alcohol consumption involves health care cost externalities, as well as social cost externalities. The extent to which it is addictive is somewhat more controversial. The desire for a glass of wine on a Friday night is a different type of addiction from the alcoholic's urge for liquor when his blood-alcohol level falls below a certain level.

Alcohol has been illegal in many countries, e.g. US and Norway, and it still is in some parts of the world. Other substances classified as narcotics are illegal in most parts of the world.

6.3.3 **Illicit drugs**

Like tobacco and alcohol, illicit drugs are characterized by their various combinations of the following features: i) detrimental effects on the user's own health, ii) negative effects on the well-being of others, and iii) their addictive character. When the aggregate effect of a substance is considered too harmful, it is no longer a 'consumer good' but a 'consumer bad'. Making it illegal is the strongest form of direct regulation available. The intention in banning a substance is that citizens should obey the law and stop demanding this 'bad good'. If they do not, illicit markets will emerge. When regulators have classified drugs as illegal, they have no remaining options for economists' favourite type of intervention, i.e. indirect regulations in the form of taxation.

Because of the penalty risks associated with market transactions, prices are driven up. Addicted users with an inelastic demand tend to finance their drugs through criminal activities. One important consideration in the issue of legalizing an illicit drug is the cost of crime.

The issue of legalizing drugs is controversial. There are three important health economic issues. First, what are the health care cost consequences? If the use of a substance is detrimental to health, and thus generates increased health care costs, again, this externality problem can be solved by levying indirect taxes on the particular drug to cover treatment costs. Second, what is the impact on other people's well-being? If the psychological reaction to the substance is one of aggression and violence, then potential victims would be best protected by banning it. Third, how addictive is the substance? If it is addictive, there is the 'soft paternalist' argument for preventing potential users from becoming hooked.

6.4 **Conclusion**

We have distinguished between two types of interventions in people's health-related lifestyle: direct regulations through the legal system, e.g. an age limit for purchasing alcohol; and indirect regulations in terms of taxes and subsidies. But what justification is there for such interventions in people's health-related choices?

There are two contrasting normative views here. One is that any activity that is detrimental to an individual's health requires some intervention from the well-informed benevolent health planner. In its extreme form this comes close to 'health fascism', or 'healthism'.[4] The other view corresponds with a crucial tenet in the paradigm of neoclassical economics, namely that the sovereign consumer is the best judge of their own welfare. While the latter view is an appealing starting point, we suggest the following issues to be considered. First, if behaviour reflects addiction and lack of foresight about the consequences on the individual's own future health, there is a 'soft paternalist' case for helping them choose differently.[5] Clearly, health-related choices are not based on preferences shaped in a vacuum, but are affected by marketing and advertisements. The more biased this type of commercially motivated information is towards unhealthy food and lifestyle choices, the stronger is the case for regulation of such information, or at least increased provision of alternative information.[6]

---

[4] See Skrabanek, P. (1994) *The death of humane medicine and the rise of coercive healthism*, Suffolk, Crowley Esmonde.

[5] Thaler and Sunstein (2008) use the concept 'libertarian paternalism'.

[6] I noticed during a visit to rural Tanzania in December 2007 that the most frequent advertising boards outside shops were for cola soft drinks and Sportsman cigarettes!

Second, if a fully informed consumer still chooses an unhealthy lifestyle, what are the health care cost implications? With private health insurance the increased expected health care costs will be internalized in the consumer's insurance premium. In a tax-financed health service, the problem can be solved by levying taxes on the risky activity. Third, are there any further costs to other members of society? If there are, there is a case for increased taxes or direct restrictions, e.g. banning smoking in public places.

Suggested reading

Nuffield Council on Bioethics (2007) *Public health: ethical issues.* London (available at http://www.nuffieldbioethics.org/).

Thaler, R. H. and Sunstein, C. R. (2008) *Nudge: improving decisions about health, wealth, and happiness.* New Haven: Yale University Press.

Lynch, J. W., Kaplan, G. A. and Salonen, J. T. (1997) Why do poor people behave poorly? Variation in adult health behaviours and psychosocial characteristics by stages of the socio-economic lifecourse. *Social Science and Medicine,* 44 (6), 809–19.

Exercises

1. Find examples of price elasticity of various types of food: healthy food such as fruit and vegetables compared with unhealthy food such as butter and sugar.

2. Explore the concepts of 'soft paternalism' and 'libertarian paternalism'. Discuss their relevance in the context of interfering in people's health-related behaviour.

3. Discuss positive and negative health consequences of legalizing some types of illicit drugs.

Part 3

Financing health care

In ordinary markets there are only two parts involved: the consumers or users who hand over money in exchange for the goods they receive, and the producers or sellers who receive the money required to cover their costs of providing the goods. In the market for health care the money flows are more complicated due to the involvement of a third party—or a 'financial intermediary'—who acts in both the role of raising revenues and the role of paying providers.

Formally, but still simply, the money flows can be expressed in terms of the 'revenue—expenditure—income' identity (see e.g. Evans, 1997). Revenues can be raised principally from four different sources: patient payments (PP), private insurance (PI), taxation for health (TH) (which also consolidates social insurance systems with payroll contributions), and voluntary donations (VD). These in sum will represent the total budget for possible expenditure, which is determined by the unit cost (C) of the different health care commodities and the quantities (Q) of each. This expenditure will always end up as income to those who provide the services. It is an indisputable fact that a given expenditure by one agent will always end up as a similarly sized income to one or more other agents, who deliver inputs such as labour, capital, and raw materials. For simplicity, and without losing general application, we can assume that everything ends up as labour income, as determined by the hours of labour (L) and the wage rate (W) per hour (which, of course, differs across the various professions involved).

This revenue—expenditure—income identity can be expressed as in Equation 7.1, in which, for simplicity, the symbols refer to vectors:

$$\begin{array}{ccccc}
revenues & \equiv & expenditures & \equiv & income \\
PP + PI + TH + VD & \equiv & C^*Q & \equiv & W^*L
\end{array} \qquad (7.1)$$

The heart of the issue here is that the identity holds as a matter of logic and simple mathematical consistency. Any change in one parameter will initiate changes in at least one other parameter. It can be either offset or balanced by a change in other parameters on the same side of the identity, or the change will lead to the same-sized total changes on each of the other two sides. An example of the former type of change is when taxes as a source of revenue are reduced but compensated for by a corresponding increase in patient payments ($\vdash\Delta TH$ | $= |+\Delta PP|$). An example of the latter is if such compensation does not take place, implying the same reduction in the other two sides of the identity, e.g. reduced quantity of health care (Q) and fewer employees in the health sector (L), i.e. $TH\downarrow \rightarrow Q\downarrow \rightarrow L\downarrow$. However, revenue reductions do not imply the same relative reductions in health care, as labour productivity may improve, with the result that unit costs fall.

There are some important distinctions that can be made between the four sources of revenue. The characteristic feature of patient payment is that it is levied ex post—after it has been established that the patient requires health care. Thus, there is a direct link between PP and C^*Q.

Private insurance premiums are, by definition, paid prior to an event, whereby the person insured purchases a guarantee of receipt of care (and attenuation of its cost), if needed. There is no cross-subsidization involved in private insurance, because the premium is based on the expected losses of the insured person.

Taxation and voluntary donations differ from the other sources of revenue in that they involve cross-subsidization; that is, the rich and/or healthy subsidize the poor and/or sick. Income taxes are normally progressive, or at least proportionate, so high income earners contribute more than low income earners to the financing of public health care. Furthermore, when there is an inverse relationship between sickness and income, high-income groups also cross-subsidize low-income groups' use of health care. In other words, high income earners contribute more than average to the funding of health care, and use less than average of the total services provided. Taxation differs from the above sources of funding in that it is compulsory.

Voluntary donations include donations to health charities, as well as any direct financial support to hospitals and health care institutions in the community, and clearly represent cross-subsidized health care.

Figure 7.1 represents the overview of the money flows between the three parts: households (citizens and patients), purchasers (government and private insurance as 'third-party payers'), and providers (primary and secondary care). Households pay for health care, directly through patient payments or voluntary donations, and indirectly through taxes and private insurance. Health care

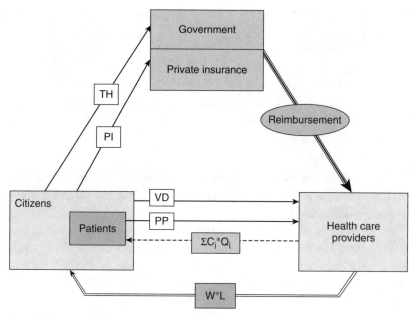

Fig. 7.1 The money flows in health care finance and provision.

providers are paid directly in terms of patient payments from patients and voluntary donations from households, or indirectly in terms of reimbursements from the third party. Patients receive health care valued at unit costs (C^*Q) from health care providers. Finally, the resources required for producing health care are delivered from the households as labour inputs, W, for which incomes (W^*L) are paid in return.

Figure 7.1 reflects Equation 7.1 in that the total revenues ($TH + PI + VD + PP$) equal expenditures (C^*Q), which again equal incomes (W^*L). However, this figure highlights something hidden in the equation: namely, the money flows that pass via the third-party payers, and the range of ways that the third parties could possibly reimburse those who provide health care. Reimbursement policies are a central part of health policy as they influence provider behaviour. Logically, there is no more money to be reimbursed than that made available through the third-party payers in terms of taxes and insurance. Part 4 of this book discusses reimbursement of providers (Chapters 10–12).

In this part of the book we will discuss the left-hand side of the identity, i.e. the different sources for raising revenues. The distinguishing characteristics of these four sources of revenues deal with: i) whether payments are made ex ante (before sickness and through a third party), or ex post (after sickness and from the patient or some donor), and ii) whether paid fully on an individual basis

	Ex ante	Ex post
No cross-subsidisation	Private health insurance	Patient payments
Coss-subsidisation	Health taxes	Voluntary donations

Fig. 7.2 A typology of revenue sources.

depending on the individual's (expected) health care use, or with any element of cross-subsidization. Figure 7.2 illustrates how the four sources fit into these different combinations:

The typology of Figure 7.2 highlights the two principal issues in health care finance: insurance and redistribution. The vertical distinction between ex ante and ex post deals with the extent of people's preferences for health insurance (their risk aversion), while the horizontal distinction deals with the extent of people's willingness to cross-subsidize their fellow citizens' use of health care.

Chapter 7 addresses the issue of health insurance, or the choice of prepayment rather than payment at the point of delivery. Chapter 8 discusses the argument for compulsory health insurance, i.e. taxation (including social insurance) rather than private health insurance. Chapter 9 discusses patient payment.

The revenue—expenditure—income identity and the three-part model in Figure 7.1 reflect a closed economy with no external flows of money for health care. In poor countries receiving health care funding from abroad, such external assistance would be channelled either directly to providers or indirectly as contributions to government or health insurance funds. Voluntary donations, be they from domestic sources or through external assistance, will not be discussed further. To most countries in the world this has relatively minor importance as a source of health care funding.

Chapter 7

Uncertainty and health insurance

A key issue in health economics is why people pay ex ante rather than ex post. There are 'welfare gains' from insurance when uncertainty is being reduced, as well as 'welfare losses' when people demand a quantity they value less than its marginal costs. Different risks of ill health across different groups of people create further inefficiencies in the market for health insurance.

We cannot insure ourselves against the risks that our house will burn down or our car will be stolen. However, we can insurance ourselves against the financial implications of such events. The same goes for health: we cannot insure ourselves against the risk of getting an illness. Health insurance, in other words, represents an insurance against the financial implications of illness, most importantly the treatment costs and lost earnings.

The characteristic of insurance schemes is the pooling of individual financial risks across all members of the pool. Risk pooling then refers to the collection and management of financial contributions so that large unpredictable individual risks become small and predictable. Participation in risk pools is either voluntary, as with private insurance, or compulsory, as with tax-funded and social insurance-funded health systems.

There are two types of uncertainty in health care that give rise to the development of such insurance schemes. First, consumers do not know if they will ever need health care. The incidence is random. Second, consumers do not know the full financial implications of illness. In order to avoid—or at least reduce—the financial uncertainties associated with future illnesses, consumers (assuming they are risk averse) take out health insurance.

People can hold three types of risk preferences. They are *risk neutral* if they have no preference between, say, the certainty of gaining a given amount and a 50% chance of gaining twice that amount. They are *risk seeking* if they prefer such a gamble, and *risk averse* if they prefer certainty. For example, would you prefer to part with €100 for certain in order to avoid a 10% risk of losing €1,000? If yes, you are risk averse. To economists, neither choice is right or wrong.

People's risk behaviour suggests that quite a few of us have different risk preferences in relation to gains compared with losses. For example, although the expected gain from (almost all) lotteries is lower than the price of the lottery ticket, people still buy such tickets, i.e. they gamble or seek risks. However, the same people may buy health or car insurance to avoid risks. This is simply because the prospects of gains activate different thoughts and emotions than do the prospects of losses: we become excited and aroused by the prospect of winning the lottery but are made anxious by the financial implications of 'health shocks'. Most people are risk averse when it comes to the financial losses associated with ill health.

7.1 **The welfare gain from insurance**

Consider an individual without insurance. If they are healthy, they enjoy wealth, W, and if they are ill, they will suffer a financial loss, L, thus resulting in $W - L$. Let the probability of illness be q; the probability of not being ill is $1 - q$. Their expected utility, $E(U)$, is their utility from wealth if they are healthy, $U(W)$, multiplied by the probability of being healthy, plus their utility from the reduced wealth if they are ill, $U(W - L)$, multiplied by the probability of their being ill:

$$E(U) = (1 - q) \, U(W) + q \, U(W - L) \tag{7.2}$$

Obviously, the smaller the probability that the illness occurs, and the smaller the expected money loss associated with the illness, the higher the expected utility.

The welfare gain from insurance can be illustrated by considering the relationship between an individual's wealth and their utility. (Recall Figure 2.2, which illustrates the crucial assumption of diminishing marginal utility of wealth.). In Figure 7.3, W on the horizontal axis represents their wealth when healthy and $U(W)$ on the vertical axis represents their utility from that wealth. $W - L$ and $U(W - L)$ show the corresponding wealth and utility, respectively, when ill. The idea of buying insurance is that the money loss, L, will be compensated for if illness occurs. The cost of this guaranteed compensation is a specified premium, p.

The premium is said to be actuarially fair if it represents the insurance company's expected payout—the size of the loss multiplied by the probability of

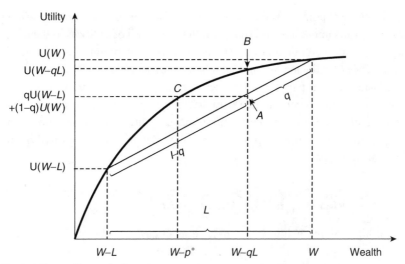

Fig. 7.3 The welfare gain from insurance.

that loss occurring, i.e. $p = qL$. When insurance is offered at actuarially fair rates to a large number of people, then the insurance company can expect to pay out the same amount in compensation as they receive in revenue from insurance premiums. Hence, actuarially fair premiums involve no profit and no cost of administering the insurance scheme.

Now compare wealth and utility with and without insurance: First, the expected wealth is the same. The left-hand side of Equation 7.3 represents wealth without insurance, and the right hand side represents wealth with insurance (when $p = qL$):

$$q\ (W - L) + (1 - q)\ W = W - qL \tag{7.3}$$

However, as can be seen from Figure 7.3, the expected utility of wealth is higher with insurance than without it:

$$q\ U(W - L) + (1 - q)U(W) < U(W - qL) \tag{7.4}$$

Thus the expected utility represents the probability-weighted average of the utility with and without loss (at point A in Figure 7.3). On the vertical axis of Figure 7.3, the utility from the insured situation reflects the point on the utility function corresponding to wealth level $W-qL$. It can be seen that the uninsured situation gives a lower level of utility. Hence, the welfare gain from insurance can be illustrated as the vertical distance from A to B between the (expected) utility without insurance and the utility with insurance.

This welfare gain to the consumer can evaporate with increased insurance premiums. The horizontal distance from point A to the intersection of the utility curve at point C indicates how much more consumers would be willing to pay for insurance and still remain at the same level of utility as in the uninsured situation. While qL $(= p)$ is the actuarially fair premium, p^* (which is larger than p) is the maximum that this consumer would be willing to pay. To the insurance company, $p^*–qL$ represents the maximum 'loading' on insurance, i.e. it is the maximum mark-up that an insurance company could charge to cover its administrative costs and to make profit. Thus, if they choose the maximum 'load factor' of $(p^* – qL) / qL$, all welfare gains are captured by the insurance company.

Would you buy health insurance?

Consider the following situation: i) you will have an income next year of €100,000, provided you stay fit and healthy, ii) you face a probability of getting ill of 1 / 6 (like throwing a dice or playing Russian roulette), and iii) if you get ill, the costs of illness next year would be €60,000, so you would be left with €40,000 in remaining income.

Your expected lost income is then 1/6* €60,000 = €10,000. An insurance company offers you an actuarially fair premium. This means you have the choice between:

A: buying this insurance and having an income of €90,000 whether you get ill or not;

B: gambling on a 1/6 probability of €40,000 and a 5/6 probability of €100,000.

If you choose A, it implies that you would in fact have been willing to pay *more than* €10,000 to avoid the risky scenario in B. What is the maximum you would be willing to pay in health insurance—or what is the lowest income you would accept in A—for you to be indifferent between A and B?

Say the maximum you are willing to pay is €15,000. This is then the maximum an insurance company can charge. Hence, if you take out insurance at that price, you are as (un)happy as you would have been if uninsured, i.e. your welfare gain from insurance has evaporated. The insurance company has earned a 'loading' of €5,000 on top of its expected loss of €10,000, which is a 'load factor' of 0.5, i.e. (15,000 − 10,000)/10,000.

7.1.1 The probability and the loss

Consider a low-probability illness with a large potential loss, q_1L_1, and compare it with a high-probability illness with a low loss, q_2L_2. Assume that the

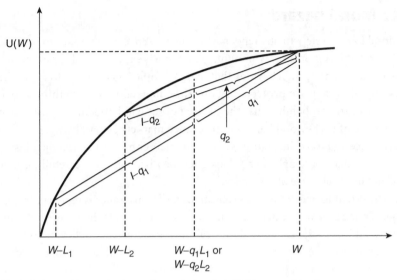

$U(W)$

$1-q_2$

q_1

q_2

$1-q_1$

$W-L_1$ $W-L_2$ $W-q_1L_1$ or W
                        $W-q_2L_2$

Fig. 7.4 The welfare gain depends on the probability*loss combination.

expected loss of the two illnesses is the same, i.e. $q_1L_1 = q_2L_2$. This means that the actuarially fair premium is the same for both illnesses. However, Figure 7.4 shows that the welfare gain from insurance is highest in the situation with the large potential loss.

The demand for insurance is at its highest when the welfare gain is highest, as illustrated by the vertical distance between the utility curve and the straight line between the two risky options. The smaller the financial loss, the smaller the welfare gains from insurance. This is intuitively appealing in that we would be less willing to take out insurance for losses that we could more easily afford. This explains situations in which insurance is not demanded.

The supply of insurance would be at its highest where the load factor is highest, as illustrated by the relative horizontal distance $(p^* - qL) / qL$. At the bottom end of the straight line between $U(W)$ and $U(W-L)$ there is no supply of insurance because the load factor is too low to cover administration costs. This explains why there is no supply of insurance contracts for illnesses with a high probability and a large loss, for example, in the case of some chronic diseases.

Hence there are efficiency reasons why insurance contracts are not specified for all types of health care: for small losses with high probabilities, there is no demand. For large losses with high probabilities, there is no supply. Below we shall see that although there are welfare gains from insurance, there may still be welfare losses associated with the consequences of insurance.

7.2 **Moral hazard**

Moral hazard refers to any tendency for the presence of insurance to increase the probability of loss or its amount. First, there is ex ante moral hazard, which refers to a change in behaviour that makes people less cautious to avoid the event when they are protected against its financial loss, something which increases the probability that the insured event will happen. There is much evidence of such moral hazard in insurance markets generally, e.g. car theft insurance and travel insurance, where customers either try to cheat their insurance company or simply do not look after their belongings as carefully as they would in the absence of insurance.

The extent to which this is a problem for health insurance is more controversial. The reason why it may be much less of a problem is the significant non-material losses associated with ill health. In general, the higher the relative importance of the non-financial utility loss associated with ill health, compared with its financial loss, the less moral hazard is involved. You do not need to pay the costs of a leg fracture, for example, but you would probably still take precautions to avoid the pain and misery of breaking your leg. Furthermore, health care is not a 'good' with intrinsic value (like a car); it is a 'necessary evil' that most of us would prefer not to consume. But still, the existence of health insurance may affect an individual's behaviour at the margin in that less effort may be made to avoid the loss.

Second, after an event has happened, we refer to it as an ex post moral hazard, reflecting the tendency to exaggerate the amount consumed above the level that would have been consumed in the absence of insurance. This may be more a problem for health insurance in that it refers to behaviour after things have gone wrong. Patients would prefer a higher level of care (and amenities) when sick than they would if they had to pay for it. Doctors, who tend to have more affinity with the patient in need than with the third party paying the bill, would be prepared to respond by recommending more resources than if the patient had to pay out of their own pocket. This supplier moral hazard exists when doctors have a great deal of discretion over the type of care they provide.

The standard—and simplest—model illustrates a situation with constant marginal costs and a downward-sloping demand curve that reflects marginal benefits (see Figure 7.5). With full insurance, a patient would prefer health care up to the point where the demand curve cuts the horizontal axis at a price of zero. Without insurance, the patient would restrict their demand where the curve cuts the marginal cost curve. The shaded triangle between the marginal cost curve and the demand curve illustrates the 'welfare loss' from insurance.

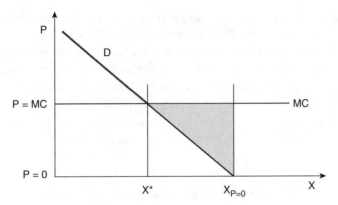

Fig. 7.5 The welfare *loss* from insurance.

Note that the size of this welfare loss crucially depends on how steep or flat the curve is. If it is steep, reflecting price-insensitive demand, there is not a problem. The flatter it is, the more problematical.

The simple policy solution to this type of ex post moral hazard is increased patient payments. The higher the co-payment (or co-insurance), the greater the reduction in the size of the welfare loss triangle. The loss completely disappears, of course, when there is no insurance. The problem with no insurance, though, is that people do not experience the welfare gains from insurance.

While maintaining the insurance system, there are various policy options to reduce ex post moral hazard. Supplier moral hazard can be reduced through contracts and treatment guidelines that attempt to restrict the choice set of the doctor in such a way that they provide services of the kind that potential patients want ex ante rather than what actual patients want ex post or what doctors themselves would want (see Part 4 of the book). Patients' ex post moral hazard can be reduced by various financial incentives such as no-claims bonuses or reductions in future insurance premiums if they do not incur costs beyond certain levels.

So far, the discussion has not taken account of real life situations that the risks of illness differ across subgroups, i.e. that people are exposed to differences in the determinants of (ill) health.

7.3 **Risks differ: actuarially fair insurance**

Let us begin by considering how a system with unregulated community rating will evaporate. Under this system, all consumers or citizens are offered the same rate that reflects the expected per capita loss over the whole community. Using C for community, the premium equals the expected loss, which is the product of the probability of the loss and the size of the loss should it occur, i.e. $p_C = q_C L_C$. However, we each have a different genetic inheritance and are exposed to different health risks (see Part 2). Consequently, each person would have their own expected loss. Imagine that n people can be located on a continuum from the lowest expected loss at one end to the highest expected loss at the other, where $q_C L_C$ represents the community average:

$$q_1 L_1 < q_2 L_2 < \dots < \mathbf{q_C L_C} < \dots < q_{n-1} L_{n-1} < q_n L_n \tag{7.5}$$

The feature of this system of community rating is that it involves redistribution ex ante, from low-risk to high-risk groups. Again, with a fixed premium, $p_C = q_C L_C$, those with lower than average risk will cross-subsidize those with higher than average risk. The further away from the community average, the larger the amount of cross-subsidy contributed or received. Clearly, all those with high risks are happy with this system (though they may of course be unhappy with their high risks).

While those with low risks might be happy with this, some might be tempted to opt out and self-insure. To the extent that they are able to signal their lower risks, an alternative insurance scheme based on individual rating will develop, in which they will be offered cheaper premiums than the current community premium. This cream-skimming of low-risk groups has some simple arithmetical implications: when low-risk individuals leave the group, the average risk (and hence premium) increases for those that remain. Persistent cream-skimming will result in each individual paying a tailor-made premium to reflect their own expected loss. Hence, under actuarially fair insurance, there is no redistribution ex ante.

High-risk individuals will have to pay high insurance premiums or else pay for health care at the point of delivery. If they cannot afford to do so (which is likely, given that high risks are often found in groups with low incomes), this is a distributional implication of actuarially fair insurance and not a market failure as such. Rather, market failure in this context relates to the problem that actuarially fair insurance is not possible due to asymmetric information.

7.4 Adverse selection

Adverse selection arises from asymmetric information about the risks faced by individuals. There is population heterogeneity in health risks due to variations in the determinants of ill health (recall Figure 5.1). If there were perfect information on how each determinant affected each one of us, it would be possible to estimate the associated individual risks and hence the actuarially fair premium for each individual. The problem is that there is asymmetric information about these risks: the individual who purchases insurance may hide information and signal false information to the agent who is selling the insurance. The lower the risk that is being signalled, the cheaper the insurance premium. Individuals may therefore claim to have a better genetic inheritance and a healthier lifestyle than are actually the case. Hence, there is an inbuilt incentive to signal false risks lower than the true risks.

The problem with actuarially fair insurance is that of signalling and identifying 'true risks'. Sellers of insurance contracts must make sure that the expected loss of a customer is not higher than the premium (plus loading). Buyers would wish to signal that they face a lower risk than they really do, in order to be offered a cheaper premium.

Since buyers may know things that the insurance company does not (or which would be too costly for the insurance company to find out), the problem for sellers is to identify and separate 'false risks' from 'true risks'. One solution is to offer contracts with deductibles (where the insured does not get compensation for losses smaller than some fixed amount) and/or co-insurance (where the insured only gets a fixed fraction of the losses covered). The market failure of this solution is that it induces self-selection: low-risk buyers will prefer contracts with high deductibles and co-insurance, while high-risk buyers will prefer more complete coverage. Consequently, the less comprehensive contracts are the cheapest because they attract low-risk buyers. In other words, the 'true low-risks' have been identified.

However, low-risk buyers might still prefer complete coverage if it were available at actuarially fair rates. But because of false signalling from high-risk buyers, this type of contract would only be offered at a rate that reflects the expected loss of the high-risk group. Hence, low-risk people are faced with the choice between partial insurance at a low rate or full insurance at an excessively high rate. In the absence of actuarially fair and full insurance, low-risk people may choose second-best partial insurance.

The more asymmetric the information is between buyers and sellers of insurance, the more severe this problem of adverse selection becomes. One way of reducing the asymmetry is for the seller to control the buyer. However, such policing and surveillance involve immense inefficiencies in terms of transaction costs. As Culyer (1989) puts it: 'Private insurance is bureaucratic and costly, requiring armies of accountants, actuaries, billers, checkers, fraud detectors, lawyers, managers and secretaries.'

Adverse selection is a consequence of the attempt at providing insurance based on individual rating, i.e. health insurance premiums are tailored to reflect individual health risks. The economic interpretation of the problem is one of inefficiency, or a market failure. This 'market failure problem' is distinctly different from the 'distributional problem'—both of which can be solved with community rating.

7.5 **Conclusion**

There is a welfare gain from health insurance because people are risk averse with respect to the financial implications of the prospect of ill health. There are effectively two main types of asymmetric information related to health insurance: adverse selection, where the asymmetry occurs before the insurance contract is made, and moral hazard, where the asymmetry occurs after the contract is made. Note, however, that moral hazard is a problem of insurance per se—irrespective of whether the premium is based on community or individual rating—while adverse selection is a problem associated only with individual rating.

We have presented two different bases for pricing health insurance: individual rating and community rating. The arguments in favour of individual rating are: i) it offers consumers a choice of contracts, ii) people have financial incentives for healthy behaviour, and iii) there is no forced cross-subsidy, i.e. it is actuarially 'fair'. The arguments against individual rating are: i) it involves adverse selection (market failure), ii) transaction costs are high due to false signalling of risks, and iii) access depends on income ('unfair'). The simplest policy solution to adverse selection, high transaction costs, and unequal access is compulsory public insurance, to which we now turn.

Suggested reading

Akerlof, G. A. (1970) The market for 'lemons': Quality uncertainty and the market mechanism. *Quarterly Journal of Economics*, 84, 488–500.

Manning, W. G. and Marquis, M. S. (1996) Health insurance: The trade-off between risk pooling and moral hazard. *Journal of Health Economics*, 15 (5): 609–39.

Robinson, J. C. (2004) Reinvention of health insurance in the consumer era. *Journal of the American Medical Association*, 291, 1880–86.

Exercises

1. Why is there more financial uncertainty for the implications of health-losses than for material losses related to e.g. house and car?

2. Imagine two types of illnesses, X and Y. For X, the probability of getting it is 50% and the cost of treatment is $200. For Y, the probability of getting it is 1%, and the cost of treatment is $10,000. There is an actuarially fair insurance on offer for each of the two. What are the rates? For which of the two illnesses would you first take out health insurance? Explain why.

3. For which types of health care do you think moral hazard is a big problem, and how would you try to solve it?

Chapter 8

Compulsory insurance

Voluntary insurance based on individual rating is costly to manage and involves inequitable access to health care. Compulsory insurance based on community rating is intended to solve these two problems.

Voluntary participation in a private risk pool offers protection against the financial costs of ill health to 'members only'. Non-members would be offered inferior services through a parallel system (or they might not be offered any health care at all). If this alternative parallel system were as good as the private option, of course there would be no demand for private insurance in the first place.

Non-participation in voluntary risk pools may reflect risk-neutral or risk-seeking preferences and hence be genuinely voluntary. However, more often it is *involuntary* due to being unable to pay the insurance premium, or because no contract is offered as a result of the individual's bad health state (chronic diseases) or high risk. Remember that in voluntary risk pools the premium is based on *individual rating*, i.e. the higher the individual's risk, the higher the premium.

Insurance based on *community rating* ignores variations in individual risks, i.e. there is no link between a person's contribution to the financing of care and their future entitlement to care. To avoid low-risk groups opting out of the system, such insurance schemes are made compulsory.

In its pure form, community rating is like a 'head tax': it is the same for all, independent of both health risks and income. A head tax is regressive (a higher proportion of income the lower the individual's income) and is therefore considered unfair. Therefore, the distribution of the financial burden is normally set either proportionate with income or progressive, meaning that the higher the individual's income, the more they contribute. In this way it represents a compulsory cross-subsidization from high income to low income groups.

Given that health and income correlate positively, there are two distinctly separate types of redistribution taking place in most compulsory health insurance schemes: i) from low-risk groups (good health) to high-risk groups (bad health), and ii) from high-income to low-income groups.

The widely stated health policy objective in many countries, of 'equal access for equal need', puts strong restrictions on how health care can be financed. Logically, if access is to be determined by need regardless of income, entitlement to care cannot be based on individual rating but must reflect some form of community rating in which contributions are made compulsory depending on ability to pay. Essentially there are two different ways of organizing revenue collection, most often referred to as social health insurance and taxation.

8.1 Social health insurance

There are—and have been—wide differences in how social health insurance (SHI) operates in practice. It was first established in Germany more than 100 years ago, and has since been established in more than 60 countries. About half of them, particularly the high income countries, have expanded to universal coverage. SHI systems are now found in many European countries (Belgium, the Netherlands, Luxembourg, France, Germany, Austria, Switzerland) and have more recently been established in many Latin American countries (see Gottret and Schieber, 2006).

Rather than describing differences, we shall focus on some general features. First, SHI is designated for group of workers or employees, and thus initially limited to the formal sector of the economy. Second, there is a direct link between being a contributing member of the scheme and being entitled to health care. Third, it is founded on the notion of *solidarity* between workers and their families, involving a high level of cross-subsidization. Fourth, the management of the system has some degree of autonomy from government.

In most cases the source of funding is payroll contribution proportional to wages, like an earmarked health tax. An alternative version of collecting the funding is one in which employers pay a fixed sum per employee, like a forced health tax per unit of labour. As such, employers are considered to bear the responsibility for maintenance of their input factors. Related to this rationale is that of reducing potential political opposition from the working class by offering workers and their families social protection in case of ill health.

The way SHI has developed to cover the whole population in high-income countries has been through state contributions financed out of general taxation. The state has thereby taken the responsibility for groups who for various reasons are not members, and has paid their premiums into the sickness funds. In some low-income countries attempts have been made to enrol groups of non-poor informal sector workers and their families, but when the contribution is a flat rate (head tax) it represents a burden for the near-poor. The bigger the informal sector, the bigger the coverage gap, and hence the slimmer the chances that SHI will lead to universal coverage[1].

SHI could be organized either in one single sickness fund or many small independent funds. They usually operate quite independent of government interference and control. Important arguments in favour of SHI are that people are more prepared to be taxed if there is a specific entitlement that accompanies the tax, and that sickness funds represent more secure funding for health care than tax-based funding. However, SHI can potentially be rather expensive to manage, particularly if many interested parties and stakeholders are involved.

8.2 Tax-financed health care

A single tax-financed public insurance appears to be the cheapest scheme when it comes to administrative costs. First, when 'health taxes' independent of individual risk are included in an existing tax system, there are no additional costs involved with revenue collection. Second, providers of health care face no costs of collecting reimbursements from the insurance companies or the sickness funds. Third, there are no costs involved in designing insurance packages for different risk groups or employment groups. Fourth, there are no advertising costs of the kind found in competitive insurance markets. Finally, as every citizen is entitled to care, there are no costs involved in checking patient eligibility.

Tax-financed health care systems that offer universal coverage are often referred to as a *national health service*, like the NHS in the UK. Such systems are found in all Nordic countries and many other high-income countries such as Italy, Spain, Portugal, Australia, New Zealand, Canada.

In low-income countries, such systems have been difficult to promote due to limited ability to raise stable and sufficient tax revenues. Tax-financed health systems are vulnerable to changes in political priorities, and may therefore be

---

[1] For a critical discussion of social health insurance and its experience in various countries, see Wagstaff, 2007.

susceptible to less secure funding than independent sickness funds. There appears to be some mixed experience as to the extent that provision reaches the poor as well as the rich. The insufficient revenue base in poor countries often results in limited service provision that extends to the rich and middle-class urban population only. And when patient co-payment is introduced as a combined source of funding, poor people are deterred from the system.

One concern among many economists is that tax financing has its own inbuilt inefficiencies in that it distorts the labour market. The higher the tax rate, the less labour supplied. Of course, the magnitude of this problem critically depends on the elasticity of labour supply (see Chapter 10), and is something that must be compared with the costs associated with the alternative ways of financing health care.

While there may be efficiency losses associated with raising tax revenues, there is one important gain associated with having *one* purchaser of health care. When negotiating with providers of care, a single purchaser will exert monopsony power (i.e. one buyer, many sellers) and may thereby achieve lower prices than in markets with many buyers. This is of course to the benefit of taxpayers, but may be less popular among health care personnel who would generally have lower salaries than in markets in which there was more than one purchaser of their services.

Tax-financed health care is often interpreted as a system that simultaneously involves both *public provision* and *public financing* of health care. This is wrong. Consider Figure 8.1. This comes from the field of public economics and illustrates the important distinction between finance and provision when discussing the public—private mix.

The vertical choice is essentially a normative one. It depends on the policy objectives regarding the principles upon which health care should be distributed. If this is 'equal access independent of income', there is a strong case against private finance. However, for the types of services for which it is accepted that

		Finance	
		Public	Private
Provision	Public	1	2
	Private	3	4

Fig. 8.1 The public—private mix in finance and provision.

access could depend on income, society might accept to move to the right of the vertical bolded line of Figure 8.1.

The horizontal choice is more about finding the best 'means to an end'. It crucially depends on which types of ownership, organization, and regulation will produce services of specified qualities in the least costly way. There are strong political views and traditions here, where 'leftists' tend to believe that the public sector is better able to provide quality services at low cost, and 'rightists' tend to believe that the private sector is best. Political discussions of the various attempts to privatize a public health service can be set within the framework of Figure 8.1. They deal either with the privatization of finance (a horizontal move from box 1 to box 2) or with the privatization of provision (a vertical move from box 1 to box 3). Hence, the question of tax-financed health care is completely separate from the question of public provision of health care.

8.3 Comparing three insurance systems

Table 8.1 sets out some key characteristics of three different health insurance systems. Most importantly, they differ in terms of three Cs: costs, coverage, and choice. Private health insurance is the most costly one to manage.[2] Coverage is limited to people who have taken out insurance, but the choice to do so is of course voluntary. The contrasting system is taxation: it is cheap, it involves universal coverage, but it is compulsory. The individual has to emigrate to avoid it!

Social health insurance lies between the two contrasting systems, but in practice is quite similar to tax-funded health care on two crucial issues. First, there is no link between size of the individual's contribution and their expected use of health care. Hence, the inefficiencies in the labour market associated with direct taxation would be the same, no matter whether some part of the compulsory taxation is 'earmarked' or not. Second, in high-income countries SHI has developed to *universal coverage* through top-up tax-financed contributions to the sickness funds from the state to cover non-member groups outside the workforce.

8.4 Conclusion

The characteristics of the systems described in Table 8.1 go to prove that we cannot have it all. A tax-financed system that is cheap to manage and offers

---

[2] US health care administration costs are 31% of total expenditures (Morris *et al.*, 2007).

Table 8.1 Key characteristics of three different health insurance systems

	Private health insurance	Social health insurance	Taxation
Cost of managing the system (revenue collection and determining access)	Expensive	From quite expensive to quite cheap	Cheap
Coverage	Limited	Formal sector only (or extended to universal)	Universal
Choice of participation	Voluntary	Compulsory for all in the formal sector	Compulsory
Cross-subsidization	No	Across other members of the formal sector	Yes
Source of funding	Individual premiums	Payroll tax	Direct and indirect taxes
Contributions based on	Health risks	Income	Income and consumption
Access based on	Income	Needs	Needs
Secure funding	Yes, increased costs → increased premiums	Yes, earmarked to sickness funds	Depends on political system
Link between size of own contribution and own expected use	Yes	No	No

universal coverage is controversial because it is compulsory and involves forced cross-subsidization from the rich and healthy to the poor and sick. The infringements in personal freedom—there is no choice between alternative insurance schemes and it involves increased taxation—may explain why this type of health insurance is sometimes referred to as 'socialized medicine'.

While the table describes separate stylized systems, in practice one system might well coexist with another. This is often the case with private health insurance, which emerges as an option to supplement collective systems. Its relative importance varies a lot between countries. The better the public system, the less demand there is for the private alternative. When private health insurance is the default system, as in the USA, there are tax-financed systems intended for those groups who would not be included in the private scheme. Even so, about 50 million of the 300 million US population have no health insurance—neither private nor covered by publicly funded systems. When in need of health care, these people would have to pay out of their own pockets—if they can.

So called out-of-pocket payments are the payments that patients have to pay at the point of delivery. No matter which health insurance system, all countries have some elements of patient payment. It is to these that we now turn.

Suggested reading

Gottret, P. and Schieber, G. (2006) *Health financing revisited: A practitioner's guide.* Washington DC: The World Bank.

Wagstaff, A. (2007) *Social health insurance re-examined.* WPS 4111. Washington DC: The World Bank (available at www.worldbank.org).

Mossialos, E., Dixon, A., Figureras, J. and Kutzin, J. (ed.) (2002) *Funding health care: Options for Europe.* Buckingham: Open University Press (see in particular Chapter 2; available at http://www.euro.who.int/document/e74485.pdf).

Exercises

1. The Netherlands have a unique health insurance system. Read about it and discuss it in relation to the three systems in Table 8.1.

2. In which institutional settings would you recommend social health insurance rather than tax-financed health care?

3. What is the biggest problem with 'socialized medicine' (tax financed): no freedom of choice, moral hazard, or other issue?

Chapter 9

Patient payment

In all countries patients pay for some types of health care,
in full or in part. This chapter discusses various types of patient
payments, their distributional effects, and the policy option of
applying *negative* patient payments to increase the utilization
of some types of health care.

The relative importance of patient payments as a source of funding differs a
lot between countries—from as low as 10% or 15% in Northern Europe
to more than 50% in poor countries. The high share in poor countries
could be explained by their lack of institutional arrangements to organize a
'financial intermediary' that collects and manages funds for risk pooling and
redistribution.

There are two kinds of somewhat rhetorical health policy arguments in
favour of more patient payments: i) 'the public purse cannot afford to pay for
all health care', and ii) 'unnecessary demand will be deterred when people pay
for themselves'. While the second argument makes sense theoretically (moral
hazard), the 'public purse cannot afford' argument is a strange one. Remember
Figure 8.1 illustrating that *all* revenues for health care expenditures originate
from households. So if patients can afford to pay through patient payment,
they can also afford to pay through increased taxation. Thus, while politically
unpopular, the logical solution to the underfunding argument is to increase
taxation.

A more fruitful approach to patient payment is to consider it as the preferred
residual way of financing health care. Remember the two reasons for free health
care: insurance (Chapter 7), and redistribution (Chapters 3 and 4). Hence,
when there is *no welfare gain* from insurance, and *no externality* in health care

use that triggers further redistribution from fellow citizens, the individual has to pay out of their own pocket at the point of delivery.

The most extensive study on the effects of patient payments was carried out in the USA more than 20 years ago. This was the Rand Health Insurance Experiment (Manning *et al.*, 1987). Some key findings were that: i) co-payment reduces the total quantity demanded, ii) demand for unnecessary health care was *not* reduced any more than the demand for necessary health care, and iii) demand was reduced more among poor people than rich people, and particularly among the children of poor people.

9.1 **The third party or the patient pays**

In principle, for every type of health care we might come to need, we would choose either to take out insurance or not. If people have taken out insurance for a particular type of care, there is no patient payment. If they have *not* insured, they are faced with payment should they come to use that type of care. The principle is simple.

But in fact, it is not that simple: if there are sufficient positive externalities involved to evoke cross-subsidization from other members of society to cover the full costs, then there will still be no patient payment. If the cross-subsidies are *less* than the costs of treatment, then, as Figure 3.2 showed, there is a case for positive patient payment. However, there might still be a simple transaction cost argument for avoiding patient payment for a particular type of health care, namely, if the administrative costs involved in collecting an optimal price exceed the revenues that would be generated.

In practice, people do not take out single item insurance contracts for every type of health care they could possibly come to need. Rather, insurance contracts include whole bundles of health care, some of which might not have been chosen by some customers. Hence, the sensible solution might well be to prefer co-insurance on some subsets of health care.

Within a tax-financed NHS scheme, it is controversial to decide which services should be provided free and which should *not* be included but instead be paid in full. Nevertheless, in most countries we find whole subsets of health care that patients have to pay in full, e.g. dental care for the adult population in Norway.

9.2 **Co-payment, co-insurance, co-funding, cost sharing**

When patient payment is being referred to as co-payment, co-insurance, or co-funding, it means that a third-party payer is also involved in the financing. 'Cost sharing' means that patients are sharing the costs with those who subsidize them.

If the co-payment is a fixed charge beyond which the third party pays the remainder, there is an incentive for the provider to increase the price: a higher price will *not* reduce demand but increases the income received from the third party.

If the co-payment is a variable charge on top of a fixed contribution from the third party, the incentive for the patient is to be cost conscious. Such pricing policies can be observed in pharmaceuticals in some countries: the third party refunds a price equal to the cost of the most cost-effective generic drug. Thus, if the patient prefers a more expensive alternative, they must pay the additional cost out of their own pocket. A scheme whereby the third party pays an initial fixed sum and the patient pays everything above this is the reverse of the principle of deductibles, whereby the patient pays some initial cost and the third party covers everything above.

9.3 **Deductibles**

The use of deductibles is a common feature of insurance contracts. Remember from Chapter 7 that the solution to the problem of adverse selection is partial insurance, i.e. the person insured is covered for financial loss beyond the level that they think they can afford. Below this level, they are prepared to pay all expenses. Above this level, the insurance company picks up the bill. In this way, there is no moral hazard below the ceiling.

The use of deductibles is a central feature of social health insurance and tax-financed health care as well as private health insurance. In Norway, when a patient's total payment for some types of primary care including GP visits and pharmaceuticals exceeds €200, the state refunds all remaining co-payments for the rest of the calendar year.

While deductibles require all patients to co-finance health care, the scheme does not necessarily affect the quantity demanded among patient groups who are frequent users: if a patient expects their aggregate annual co-payment to exceed the ceiling, they know that their marginal co-payment will be zero; so the existence of a positive price on the first units purchased does not affect total demand. Hence, among frequent users of health care, the deductible operates like a 'head tax' (a uniform fixed amount per individual patient) independent of their health care utilization—and of their income.

Figure 9.1 illustrates a situation where a patient's demand is unaffected by the existence of co-payments. This is because the deductible becomes effective *before* their maximum willingness to pay for the marginal unit is equal to the co-payment rate, p_{CP}. The patient pays for their utilization up to the quantity, X_{DED}, at which point the deductible, $(p_{CP}{}^* X_{DED})$ is reached. Beyond this quantity, he is faced with a zero price and, thus, demand, $X_{p=0}$.

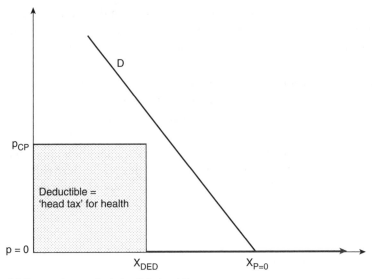

Fig. 9.1 Demand exceeds deductible level X_{DED}.

Figure 9.2 shows the demand curve of another patient. This individual is poor and their demand, D_{POOR}, is compared with the demand from the patient in Figure 9.1, who happened to be rich, D_{RICH}. The key difference between the two patients is that the poor patient's maximum willingness to pay for each marginal unit is lower—and equal to p_{CP}, the co-payment rate—before the poor

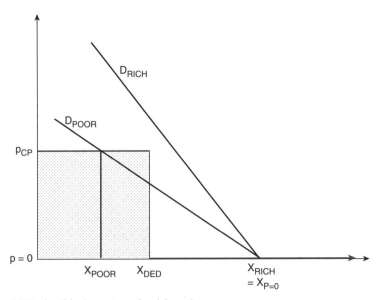

Fig. 9.2 Deductible: impact on the rich vs the poor.

patient reaches the deductible. In the absence of co-payments, both patients would have used similar quantities, $X_{P=0}$. Note the inequitable implications of this combined policy of co-payments and deductibles for the differences in utilization: the poor patient's utilization is constrained by co-payment, while the rich patient's is not. The rich patient has paid a 'head tax' (= deductible).

9.4 **Distributive implications**

A general policy lesson from patient payment schemes is that the reduction in the quantity demanded is higher among poor people than rich people, i.e. poor people have more elastic demand for health care. Consider now two children; Richard, born to rich parents, and Poorard, born to poor parents.[1] They suffer from the same disease and have an identical need for health care, e.g. paediatric consultations. In Figure 9.3 the demand curve of Poorard's parents is flatter than that of Richard's parents, indicating that Poorard's utilization is more sensitive to the price of care. When $p = 0$, they have identical utilization at $X_{p=0}$. The 'problem' here is that they both value the marginal units lower than the marginal costs, as illustrated by the 'welfare loss' triangles (the area between the MC curve and the demand curve, to the right of the intersection between $MC = D$). Note that this 'excess demand' is bigger for Poorard than for Richard.

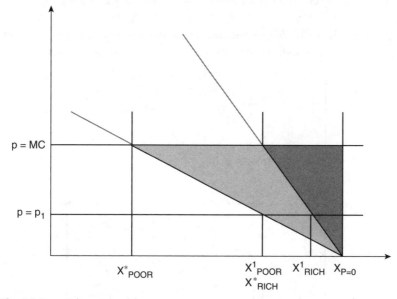

Fig. 9.3 Demand: poor vs rich.

---

[1] This example is inspired by an exercise provided by Uwe Reinhardt (1998).

If some co-payment, $p = p_1$, is introduced in order to deter excess demand, Poorard's utilization will be reduced to X^1_{POOR} and Richard's to X^1_{RICH}. If payments were to increase further in order to get rid of *all* welfare losses, i.e. where they equal marginal costs, then Poorard's optimal utilization would be X^*_{POOR} and Richard's X^*_{RICH}. Note that this optimal quantity for Richard is exactly the quantity which Poorard had when the price was p_1, which was *not* considered optimal for Poorard, simply because Poorard's parents value this marginal unit below its marginal costs, while Richard's parents value it at its marginal costs. In other words, given that the optimal quantity is defined to be that where the marginal valuation equals the marginal costs, it is 'correct' that Poorard gets less health care than Richard. So what is considered *excess demand* in this context bears no resemblance to whether it is a *medically* unnecessary utilization, but rather to people's insufficient monetary valuations, which depend on their *ability to pay*.

9.5 **Negative patient payments**

When positive prices work in the sense that they *deter* demand, so should negative prices work in the sense that they *attract* demand. And given that poor patient groups are more sensitive to prices than are rich groups, they will increase their demand more if receiving some monetary premium for seeking health care.

Consider Figure 9.4, with a horizontal marginal cost curve, a demand curve D_I that shows users' individual valuations (their private benefits) of increasing

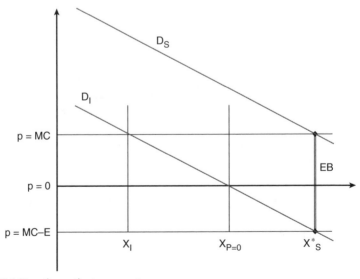

Fig. 9.4 Negative patient payment.

units, and a social demand curve D_S that shows society's total valuation (social benefits) of increasing units, i.e. the individual valuation *plus* the valuation of the positive externalities, or what in Chapter 3 we called external benefits, *EB*, involved in the use of this particular health care: $D_S = D_I + EB$.

Three alternative quantities are shown: X_I is the quantity consumed if patients were to pay everything out of pocket, $X_{p=0}$ is the quantity consumed if it was provided free, and X^*_S is the *optimal quantity* consumed, i.e. where society's marginal valuation equals marginal cost. In order to reach this optimal quantity, users would have to receive a premium equal to the marginal costs minus the valuation of external benefits: $p = MC - EB$. Hence, as for health care involving large positive externalities, there is nothing in theory to suggest that such health care should be provided at zero price. For example, negative patient payments on some types of vaccination may prove to be an effective way of reaching the target population.

Of course, negative patient payments represent a health care *cost*, as opposed to (positive) patient payments, which are a source of *revenue*. The implication is that the funding of such a scheme requires more money to be collected from other sources, e.g. higher taxation.

9.6 **Autonomous consumer or compliant patient**

For almost all types of health care, the law of the downward-sloping demand curve holds: increased price → reduced quantity demanded. Given the above argument that 'unnecessary demand will be deterred when people pay for themselves', the question is whether the demand for *unnecessary* health care is *more* sensitive to price increases than is the demand for *necessary* health care. There is mixed evidence here. When degree of necessity is measured by the expected improvement that an intervention may have on people's health, people appear to be uninformed regarding which type of health care is more necessary than another, in that the price elasticity is quite independent of how effective the particular type of health care is.

What does seem to be the case is that if a doctor has recommended a particular type of health care, the price has less deterrent effect than for those types of health care we use *without* consulting a doctor. Figure 9.5 illustrates the process from the role of 'autonomous consumer' to 'compliant patient'. First, for whatever reason, an individual wonders if they should go and see the doctor. If they do so, *demand* for health care can be observed. The doctor then assesses the individual's *needs* and gives their recommendations. If these require the individual to use health care (e.g. referrals, drugs), and the individual takes the doctor's advice, they can be observed to demand the type of health care recommended. However, since demand is a concept associated

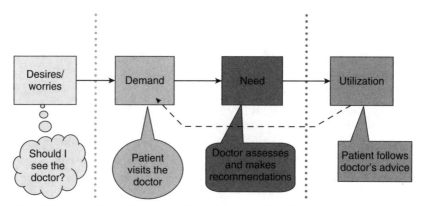

Fig. 9.5 Patient-initiated demand vs doctor-initiated utilization.

with the choices of autonomous consumers (in isolation from suppliers), rather than something that is initiated from an agent, *utilization* is used here to distinguish it from demand. The doctor may also recommend that the individual returns for a later consultation 'to see how things are going', and if so, the doctor initiates—or *induces*—demand. (The concept of 'supplier-induced demand' is discussed in the next chapter).

The dotted vertical lines of Figure 9.5 illustrate two types of barriers that patient payment represent, either to deter patient-initiated demand, or to deter what in fact is a doctor-initiated utilization. The Rand study on the quantity effect of co-payments showed that the price elasticity of demand was less elastic for hospital care than for other types of care, which could be explained by the fact that most hospital care is recommended by a doctor.

9.7 **Conclusion**

Theory and practice show that patient payments reduce the demand for health care, and that reductions are larger among the poor than the rich. Furthermore, practice shows that patient payments do not make us reduce demand for unnecessary health care more than for necessary care, something which can be explained by the fact that patients are uninformed: we simply do not know what is more necessary. This is why we seek a doctor's advice.

To protect us from financial loss following the need for large quantities of health care, deductibles are a common feature of most insurance plans, i.e. a ceiling beyond which patients are not charged any further payments. Interestingly, people who expect to use health care at the level where their aggregate co-payments *exceed* the ceiling know they will face a zero price on their marginal health care consumed. Hence, co-payments will have no deterrent effect on frequent user groups. Rather, the deductible operates like a 'head tax' on these patient groups. It is only when annual health care utilization involves aggregate co-payments *below* the ceiling that co-payments are effective in reducing utilization. Given that most of us have health care consumption below this level, co-payments do have the effect of reducing our health care utilization.

The quantity reduction of co-payments is lower for the types of health care that are recommended by doctors, simply because patients in general comply with doctors' advice. So if the policy aim with co-payments is to combat unnecessary utilization, it seems strange to put the incentive on the patient as opposed to the doctor. Among other things, the next part of this book looks at doctors' remuneration.

Suggested reading

Manning, W. G. *et al*. (1987) Health insurance and the demand for medical care: evidence from a randomized experiment. *The American Economic Review*, 77, 3: 251–77.

Folland, S., Goodman, A. C. and Stano, M. (2007) *The Economics of Health and Health Care*. New Jersey: Pearson Education (see Chapter 9).

Reinhardt, Uwe (1998) Abstracting from distributional effects, this policy is efficient. In *Health, Health Care and Health Economics: Perspectives on Distribution* (ed. M. L. Barer, T. E. Getzen and G. L. Stoddarts). Chichester: Wiley.

Exercises

1. For which types of health care would you recommend patient payments, and for what theoretical reasons?

2. Discuss a policy that makes deductibles income dependent in order to reduce the inherent problem of inequitable health care utilization.

3. What is positive about negative patient payments?

Part 4

Paying health care providers

We now turn to the money flows from third-party payers to providers, i.e. the reimbursement arrow of Figure 7.1. Apparently things were simpler in the old days: in tax-funded systems, government would simply divide its health care budgets across hospitals. If waiting lists occurred, hospital managers could blame politicians for not having allocated enough money. In private health insurance systems, providers would bill the insurer for the costs incurred. If these were too expensive, hospital managers could argue that everything was needed.

While there are many ways to pay providers, the choice set of purchasers may be constrained by the ways in which revenues are collected. Remember the 'revenue—expenditure—income' identity: the total sum of money that providers receive from third-party payers cannot exceed the revenues that the same third party collects from households. Thus, moving towards activity-based funding, which often implies increased expenditures, would require some associated discretion in raising more money.

An important feature of health policy reforms in countries with tax-funded health services has been the various attempts at drawing a split between purchasers and providers. Hospitals no longer have to be publicly owned and receive fixed budgets from government. Instead, their budgets might come to depend on their activity, and they might even become privately owned. In private insurance systems, there has been a change from retrospective reimbursement of costs to prospective payments.

The key distinction in the various ways of paying providers is whether payment is activity based or not. Hospitals can receive fixed budgets independent of activity, or be reimbursed depending on how many patients they treat.

General practitioners can be salaried independent of their activity or be remunerated based on activity measures, usually fee for service or fee per patient (capitation). The question then is which system or combination of systems to choose.

The underlying rationale behind activity-based health care funding is the belief that financial incentives will make providers become more efficient, i.e. that external rewards motivate increased efforts. It is a type of incentive contracting, whereby a principal (health care purchaser) will induce and reward certain behaviour by the agent (health care provider).

While there is evidence that activity-based reimbursement improves cost-efficiency, there are other negative effects that make it a controversial health policy. The problem is similar to that with medicine: in addition to the intended effects, there might be unintended side effects. In a recent review of performance-related pay in health care, Mannion and Davies (2008) contend that 'Evaluation of pay for performance initiatives has not kept pace with the rush to implement them', and cite studies that have found either no effect or negative effects of introducing financial incentives.

In addition to the aim of efficiency within each of the two major levels of provision, there are various ways in which overall efficiency of the delivery system can be improved through better integration between provider levels. Many economists have an affinity with the idea of 'internal markets' and many policy makers are thrilled by the rhetoric of 'The money should follow the patient.'

This part of the book discusses the various ways in which providers at the two key health care provider levels can be paid, how to remunerate general practitioners in primary care, and how to reimburse hospitals in specialized care. Given the characteristic feature of patient flows through the delivery system, a brief chapter is included on the importance of integrating the different health care provider levels—not only primary and secondary care, but prescriptive medications and referrals to tertiary care as well.

Chapter 10

Primary care

The most widely used models for paying general practitioners are: fee for service, capitation, and salary. Each scheme has its pros and cons, which explains why we observe blended remuneration systems in practice.

The focus here will be on general practitioners (GPs)—sometimes called primary care physicians (PCPs)—outside hospitals, who work in single practices or jointly with other doctors. In larger practices, other health care personnel may be involved, such as nurses or midwives. These groups would normally be salaried.

The key distinction is whether remuneration varies with activity or not. If not, the practitioner receives a salary, which of course will depend on the number of hours worked but will be independent of their activity during these hours. In addition, the GP practice may receive some allowances to cover fixed costs based on e.g. local cost variations or recruitment problems.

Activity-based remuneration is essentially of two types: i) capitation, i.e. determined by the number of patients on the list, and ii) fee for service, i.e. determined by which services are provided during consultation. Such activity-based compensation can be seen as an incentive contract between a principal (third-party payer) and an agent (primary care physicians): when there is asymmetric information and hence it is costly for the principal to observe the agent's performance, the principal would seek to design payment contracts that motivate the agent to become more productive, or—within multitask jobs—to perform more of those tasks that the principal would prefer to have done. Interestingly, however, activity-based remuneration in general practice is not something that is always initiated by the principal; doctors themselves seem to prefer elements of such payment schemes.

10.1 **Fee for service**

Fee for service (FFS) is defined as a payment mechanism in which a provider is paid for each individual service rendered to a patient. FFS has the dual purpose of covering the costs that the task incurs on the practice, but also of being a financial incentive for the doctor (as agent) to perform more of the tasks that the purchaser (as principal) would like the doctor to do. To fulfil this latter purpose, the preferred tasks would be remunerated at a higher rate per unit of the doctor's effort.

A general lesson from performance-related pay schemes is that the agent puts more time, attention, and effort into those tasks that are being measured and rewarded—and consequently less effort elsewhere. General practice is a genuinely multitask job. There are huge variations in symptoms, and patients with a given symptom vary in terms of how they would like to be treated during consultation. As such, FFS is an immensely sophisticated fee structure, more complicated than most other performance-related pay schemes.

Fees can either be paid out of pocket by the patients who use the services or be reimbursed from a third party. In some countries, patients pay a fixed co-payment for consultation, while the services provided during consultation are reimbursed from the third-party payer.

The more services provided, the higher the income. A general finding of the effect of this remuneration system is that it makes participating doctors provide more services than their salaried equivalents. The controversial issue is whether this in general is a good thing, and particularly whether FFS makes doctors provide too many services.

Given the asymmetric information between doctors and patients, doctors—as suppliers of health care—have much discretion in influencing patients' demand. Hence, when patients' demand for doctors' services directly determine the latters' income, doctors have an incentive to induce demand—particularly if their current income is below what they consider to be their 'target income'. Bearing in mind the discussion in the previous chapter on demand vs utilization (see Figure 9.4), the term utilization should be used rather than demand for the type of health care consumption that is preceded by a doctor's recommendation. However, the health economics literature does not usually make this conceptual distinction. Hence the concept 'supplier-induced demand' instead of 'supplier-induced utilization'.

10.1.1 **Supplier-induced demand**

The heated issue is whether doctors induce more demand than the patient would prefer, had the patient had the same level of information. Supplier-induced demand (SID) refers to the extent to which a doctor provides or

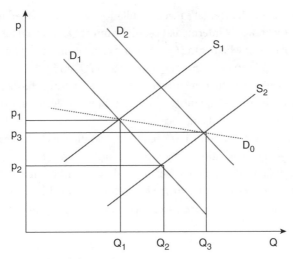

Fig. 10.1 Supplier-induced demand.

recommends medical services beyond what the patient would have chosen if they had available the same information and knowledge as the doctor. Few issues in the health economics literature have generated more interest and controversy than SID—in terms of both theoretical debates and breadth of empirical investigations.[1]

Consider a market for primary care physician services, as shown in Figure 10.1. Initially, there is the general case of a downward-sloping demand curve, D_1, and an upward-sloping supply curve, S_1. Where these two curves intersect, the market is being cleared in a quantity Q_1 and a price p_1. Imagine then an increased supply of doctors, something which will shift the supply curve to the right, S_2. The new equilibrium would be at Q_2 and p_2. This is of course appreciated by patients who face a lower price, but unfortunate for doctors who experience a drop in their income. As with other groups of people faced with the prospect of an income drop, we would assume that doctors react rather than relax. How do they do so—by inducing demand? If so, this is illustrated by a shift in the demand curve, D_2, to the new equilibrium at Q_3 and p_3. This is unfortunate for patients who face a higher price (though lower than initially in this figure), but fine for doctors who receive a higher income than they would have done without inducing the demand.

....

[1] When the tribal language is one of variation over 'supply' and 'demand', it is easy to understand why a concept that merges these two mantra words appears to have some arousal effects on many economists!

In practice, these changes take place simultaneously, and it is therefore hard to observe the theoretically intermediate equilibrium at Q_2 and p_2. The controversial empirical issue is whether the true demand curve is the dotted one, D_O, passing through the observed points (Q_1 and p_1) and (Q_3 and p_3), or the curve D_2. One crucial issue is whether doctors have the power to shift the demand curve further out in the price—quantity space, and how the eventual extent of this inducement could be tested empirically.[2]

The main macro test to date has been to look at the effect of a change in the population—physician ratio on doctors' fees and the use of services. Typically this is undertaken by using cross-sectional data. As different areas may produce different utilization rates or fee levels for reasons other than physician supply, data on other factors are also used to control for potential confounding factors.

The hypothesis is that doctors, behaving entirely rationally, respond to an increase in the supply of doctors by generating greater demand for their services to maintain their target level of income. There is plenty of evidence to suggest that there is a positive relationship between supply of doctors and the use of medical services. However, this is not necessarily a causality, since doctors might be attracted to areas with many illnesses and health care needs. The evidence for the relationship between the supply of doctors and fees is less conclusive.

Micro tests of SID concentrate on doctors' responses to financial incentives by looking at how doctors respond to fee controls or to a change in their method of remuneration. The hypothesis being tested is that both fee controls and a change in methods of remuneration will lead to a change in the quantity of services being provided as doctors attempt to maintain their target income. Such 'natural experiments' do not have many of the drawbacks of the macro tests, e.g. typically there is better-quality data and fewer confounding factors.

---

2 One of the world's most prominent health economists, Victor Fuchs, published a unique editorial in the *Journal of Health Economics* in response to an article entitled 'Induced demand—can we ever really know its extent?'on the empirical problem of detecting SID. Fuchs saw a parable in a story of a Frenchman who hired a private detective to find out if his wife was unfaithful: '. . . a few days later the detective came and gave his report: "One evening when you were out of town I saw your wife get dressed in a slinky black dress, put on perfume, and go down to the local bar. She had several drinks with the piano player and when the bar was closed they came back to your house. They sat down in the living room, had a few more drinks, danced, and kissed." The Frenchman listened intently as the detective went on: "Then they went upstairs to the bedroom, they playfully undressed one another, and got into bed. Then they put out the light and I could see no more." The Frenchman sighed: "Always that doubt, always that doubt."' (Fuchs, 1986).

These tests provide compelling evidence of physicians changing their level and/or type of services provided in line with predictions from the target income hypothesis. Depending on the fee structure, they could have incentives to provide more services internally in the GP practice (e.g. some simple blood tests), more referrals to specialists and hospital services (e.g. X-rays), and, finally, recall visits (e.g. 'Come and see me again in three weeks' time.').

The normative debate about SID has dealt with the extent to which we can accuse doctors of doing such bad things for patients—since almost by implication SID is a bad thing. Whether or not it really is has a simple analytical answer: namely, whether the demand has been shifted to the right of the point where the initial (and assumed autonomous) demand curve hits the horizontal quantity line, i.e. where marginal benefit to the patient equals marginal costs (= 0). If it has not, this partial model suggests that the doctor has not done anything morally wrong to the patient. Whether or not SID is morally wrong for society depends on whether or not demand has been pushed to the right of the point at which society's valuation of marginal benefits is lower than marginal costs, something which is more likely to happen.

It is reasonable to conclude that some demand inducement exists—we might not be able to see it but we can certainly smell it and taste it! The shift in the demand curve is symptomatic of an imperfect agency relationship arising out of asymmetric information, which gives the doctor some discretion in their decisions, and personal transactions, which means that the doctor can persuade the patient to trust those decisions. This is despite the fact that most health professionals are motivated by a moral duty towards their patients, something which together with the code of medical ethics—non-maleficence, beneficence, autonomy, and justice—will act as powerful constraints on the income-maximizing behaviour.

While SID has been dealt with here as something related to fee for service as a remuneration system for GPs, it may well appear in other settings in which there is a direct link between the amount of services provided and doctors' income, such as some types of specialist care. Note that what is important for the analyses of SID is that doctors' income depends on the amount of services they provide. Who pays the fee (patients or third party) is not the concern here, though it is likely that doctors are more tempted to induce demand when the third party picks up the bill.

10.2 Capitation

Capitation is a remuneration system that breaks the link between payment and amount of service provided, and hence reduces doctors' incentives to induce demand for their services. Capitation has two separate features. First, it is an organization model, referred to as a list patient system which gives each citizen the right to have their own GP. There are good arguments for sticking to a long term-relationship with your GP rather than shopping around. A family doctor knows the health history of their patient and would therefore have a better informational basis for setting a precise diagnosis, as well as recommending a treatment that may correspond with the patient's preferences. Capitation has the potential for greater continuity of care, and more loyalty between doctor and patient. As with other relationships, it takes time to establish trust: patients trust their family doctor more than they trust someone new. All this explains why a well functioning list patient system appears to be popular both among GPs and patients.

Second, capitation is a payment mechanism in which the GP receives a fixed fee for each person registered on their list, so their income depends on the size of the patient list. Note that the remuneration model does not follow from the organization model! A list patient system can operate with family doctors but with GPs still being paid through fee for service or salaries.

The incentive under capitation is to compete for patients. However, in practice, the length of the list is normally regulated, with an upper maximum of around 2,000 patients. Once doctors reach their threshold number, the incentive to attract more patients disappears. There remains an inbuilt incentive to 'cream-skim', i.e. to selectively attract healthy patients rather than less healthy patients, and even to dump time-consuming patients by behaving in ways that lead them to choose a different GP. The solution to cream-skimming is risk-adjusted capitation in accordance with the patient mix, so that more weight is given to patients with greater needs.

Another incentive under capitation is to increase referrals, and hence shift costs to specialists and hospitals. Clearly, internally provided services incur costs in a practice. It is cheaper for the GP to 'free-ride' by sending patients to specialists where they can obtain the services they need. Furthermore, when patients have the option to change GP, there is a danger of losing patients if the doctor is not sufficiently prepared to meet patients' requests. Hence, there is an inbuilt incentive to 'try to keep the customer satisfied' by acceding to requests for sick leave or agreeing to unnecessary referrals to hospitals for further tests such as X-rays. As such, primary care doctors become less concerned with their role as gatekeeper. Finally, something which would be considered a positive effect of capitation is the incentive for greater preventive activity, since healthy patients seek doctors more rarely.

GPs who do not reach the maximum number of patients on the lists, or who have stated that they are prepared to enrol more patients, will have an incentive to provide more services for their current patients—if there is a blended remuneration system including fee for service. In other words, lost capitation income might be compensated by increased income from providing more services to fewer patients.[3]

10.3 **Salary**

While there are many things that affect an individual's choice of whether to work, the wage rate is certainly a crucial variable and therefore an important incentive device. As to the choice of how much to work, the conventional perception seems to be that the same causal relation exists as for the choice of whether to work, namely that increases in the wage rate will always attract a person to work more. However, this is not necessarily the case.

Consider an individual who faces a time constraint. During a given time period (a year, a week, or a day), a given proportion is devoted to work and the rest is leisure. The income the individual receives depends on how much they work and the wage rate. Let us assume that all other things that may affect labour supply are constant and that the only relevant goods in life are income (from which consumption goods can be purchased) and leisure. By implication, it follows that work is a bad that has instrumental value only—in terms of it being a source of income (which is unfortunately true for many people).

Now consider the situation where an individual can freely choose the number of hours worked. Except for the variables on the axes, Figure 10.2 is similar

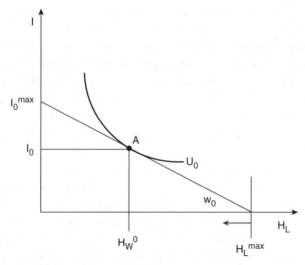

Fig. 10.2 Trade-off between income and leisure.

---

[3] For Norwegian evidence, see Iversen, 2005.

to Figure 2.7 in that it illustrates an indifference curve, U_0, a budget constraint and the optimal choice at point A, given the constraint. (A more realistic budget line would account for a minimum wage, or supplementary benefits if out of work, as well as minimum leisure time required for sleeping). The horizontal axis measures the number of hours for leisure, H_L, which has a logical maximum (only 24 hours in a day) at the intersection $H_L{}^{max}$. The vertical axis measures income, I, with a maximum income—shown at $I_0{}^{max}$. The slope of the budget line is the wage rate, w_0. Given the wage rate and the leisure—income preferences of this individual, their demand for leisure is shown by $H_L{}^0$ and their corresponding supply of labour, or working hours, becomes $H_W{}^0 = (H_L{}^{max} - H_L{}^0)$, yielding an income $I_0 = w_0{}^*H_W{}^0$.

What happens with an increase in the wage rate? Figure 10.3 illustrates this by a steeper budget line. The individual can move further out in their utility space and land at a point C, where an indifference curve, U_1, is tangential to the new budget line. There are two simultaneous effects taking place now. First, there is an income effect that follows from the fact that leisure is a 'normal good' (defined as a good for which an individual would increase their demand when their income increases, i.e. the higher the income, the more leisure they can afford), and thus the more they will demand. In isolation, this partial effect of a wage increase would imply a reduced supply of labour.

Second, there is a substitution effect that follows from the fact that leisure has become more expensive, in that the forgone income from not working an extra hour is higher, i.e. the opportunity costs of leisure have increased. This partial effect of leisure having become a more expensive good would imply less demand for it with a corresponding increased supply of labour.

In Figure 10.3, we have illustrated the two partial effects by adding a hypothetical (dotted) budget line that is parallel to the new budget line and tangential to the initial indifference curve at point B. This point is characterized by leaving the individual at their initial utility level but with the new wage rate. A real world policy that might explain this hypothetical shift would be the introduction of a poll tax (or head tax) and a wage increase that makes the individual as happy as before, i.e. they are indifferent between A and B. However, at this new point the individual works more and gets a higher income (higher than the poll tax). When this hypothetical poll tax is abolished, they move from B to C, a move that is characterized by more leisure and more income. In other words, the result of the wage increase can then be explained by a substitution effect from A to B and an income effect from B to C. Given that these two effects work in opposite directions with regard to labour supply, the question is: which effect is larger in absolute terms? Figure 10.3 illustrates

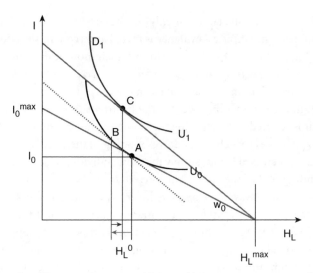

Fig. 10.3 Trade-off between income and leisure: higher wage → more work.

a situation with increased labour supply, but it is easy to draw an indifference curve whereby labour supply decreases. Find a sheet of paper and do so!

By making further increases in the wage rate, the loci of the preferred income—leisure points can be identified. These points can then be translated into a supply curve for labour, as in Figure 10.4, where the horizontal axis measures the number of working hours, H_W, and the vertical axis measures the wage rate, w. We have illustrated a backward-bending curve, whereby increases in the wage rate will lead to increased labour supply if the wage is low, but to reduced labour supply when the wage rates become very high.

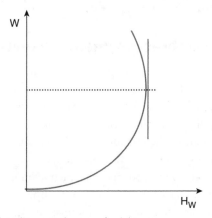

Fig. 10.4 Backward-bending supply curve for labour.

At which wage rate the labour supply curve starts to bend backwards is far from clear-cut. The empirical evidence is mixed and economists naturally disagree on this. Still, this model may help to explain how health care personnel respond to changes in their wage systems. There is evidence that people respond to reductions in the wage rate by increasing the labour supply in order to maintain a given income level. In the health economics literature, such behaviour is referred to as reflecting the 'target income hypothesis'. More generally, tax increases (which imply corresponding reductions in the wage rate) may result in increased labour supply for those individuals located at the backward-bending part of the curve. This is contrary to the conventional wisdom that income taxes always have negative incentives on labour supply.

One crucial lesson from the framework of Figures 10.2 and 10.3 is that it is the marginal wage rate that influences a person's propensity to supply an additional hour of labour. So when comparing a high base rate independently of how many hours are worked against a system with a low base rate for normal hours and increasingly high overtime rates, the latter wage package will generate a higher supply of labour. The alternative, with an increased base rate, means that income effect becomes relatively larger, and so there is the danger of hitting the backward-bending part of the labour supply curve.

The above discussion on the effect of changing salaries on labour supply has relevance beyond the current context of GP remuneration. Most other groups of health care personnel involved in primary care are salaried, and so are most hospital employees—including doctors. There are two important lessons following from the above analysis. First, increased salary does not necessarily imply that employees would work more. Second, if health care personnel are scarce and hospitals want their employees to work more hours, they should design a wage package with a low base rate and increasing overtime rates, rather than increase the base rate.

10.4 Comparing three payment systems

The three payments systems have been analysed in their standard and simplest form, with an assumption of linearity in performance and reward, i.e. a proportional increase in revenues from increases in fees, or in patients on the lists, or in working hours (until overtime rates take effect). In practice, these systems could be modified by introducing a diminishing, or even zero, marginal reimbursement when the GP has reached a certain pre-specified activity level. Capitation systems would normally have a maximum number of patients that each doctor could have on their list. There appears to be less restriction on the magnitude of service provision reimbursed under fee for service, but it is perfectly possible to introduce expenditure caps, such as in Germany for

Table 10.1 Key characteristics of three different remuneration systems in primary care

	Fee for service	**Capitation**	**Salary**
Behavioural response	Increase provision of services	Keep all patients satisfied (but not necessarily the costly ones)	'The patient in front of me shall be my only consideration'
Negative effects	Over-provision of own services Supplier-induced demand	Under-provision of own services Cream-skimming	Cost-inefficiency in primary care Waiting time
Cost control within primary care	Bad	Good	Very good
Gate keeping	Good	Bad	Good

pharmaceutical prescriptions. Other systems may yield increasing marginal reimbursement with bonuses after certain targets have been reached, such as the recent UK reform on points for clinical indicators.

Table 10.1 sums up some key features of the three remuneration systems in their pure forms. The incentive, and hence expected behavioural response, under fee for service is to increase provision of own services, whether this involves many services to few patients or few services to many patients. Under capitation, the doctor would try to keep all their patients satisfied, while under a salary system in which income does not depend on the number of satisfied patients, the doctor might choose to focus only on the patient in front of them.

The negative effects under FFS are over-provision of services, possibly even beyond a level preferred by patients. Capitation may lead to under-provision of services and even dumping of costly patients. A salary system has no financial incentive for cost efficiency. More time is spent with each patient, and less of the total time is allocated to direct patient consultation. However, when it comes to cost control and gatekeeping, a salary system appears to be the best alternative.

Fee-for-service systems are bad for cost controls at the primary care level, but good for cost control at the secondary level. GPs are paid for providing services at the primary level, rather than making referrals to secondary care. Hence, they are good gatekeepers.

What appears to be the most negative incentive effect of capitation is that it makes GPs less effective as gatekeepers. They have an incentive to reduce own costs by forwarding patients to the secondary care level. And as mentioned above, to avoid losing patients, they become too permissive in fulfilling their patients' wishes for medically unnecessary secondary care and for giving them sick-leave notes.

Interestingly, no single system emerges as best. In the absence of one theoretically optimal system, it is easy to understand why we observe so many blended systems in practice, and also why there are some quite strong regulatory measures aiming at reducing some of the negative effects within each system.

This chapter has focused on the incentives, and therefore the assumed effects, of the payment models in their pure form. The reason why we observe mixed—or blended—systems in practice is to counteract the partial negative effect of one system with the positive effect of another. In their review of the literature on capitation and incentives in primary care, Iversen and Lurås (2006) conclude by favouring a mixed-payment system of needs-adjusted capitation and fee for service. The critical issue then is which relative proportion these two elements should have.

There is no universally optimal mix of payment schemes. What may seem optimal in one country is not optimal in another. It depends on a range of other factors, most importantly the extent of non-financial regulations and secondary care. If secondary care is characterized by high capacity, activity-based funding, and no patient co-payments, the GP may be more inclined to make referrals. So when the gatekeeper role is vulnerable, capitation becomes problematic. If there is little regulation in terms of clinical guidelines or activity standards, fee for service may lead to over-provision and even SID, while salary systems may lead to inefficiencies.

One recent systematic review on the impact of different methods of payment (fee for service, capitation, salary, and mixed systems) on the clinical behaviour of primary care physicians concluded that: 'There was considerable variation in study setting and the range of outcomes measured. FFS resulted in more primary care visits/contacts, visits to specialists and diagnostic and curative services but fewer hospital referrals and repeat prescriptions compared with capitation. Compliance with a recommended number of visits was higher under FFS compared with capitation payment. FFS resulted in more patient visits, greater continuity of care, higher compliance with a recommended number of visits, but patients were less satisfied with access to their physician compared with salaried payment.' (http://www.cochrane.org/reviews/en/ab002215.html)

So the empirical evidence is supportive of what theory predicts, in terms of the direction of the effects. However, the strengths of the effects may not always be sufficiently large to outweigh the transaction costs involved in running a sophisticated blended remuneration system and the possible existence of some negative side effects.

10.5 **Conclusion**

While criticizing doctors is popular amongst economists, we do not believe that doctors are a priori any worse than other professions with the same length of education (and/or status). But we do pause to wonder why there is so much variety in the wage systems of doctors, where each system is judged according to how effective its financial incentives are in making doctors act in accordance with stated policy objectives. Most other professionals are salaried and are assumed not to need any additional financial incentives to make them work appropriately.

The founder of the British National Health Service, Aneurin Bevan, said that 'if you want to send a message to a doctor, you must write it on a cheque'. But often people behave in ways we expect them to. So if we design a sophisticated payment system in which a professional's income depends on every move they make, doctors may easily end up with a selfish pecuniary eye on every clinical decision. Alternative incentives lie in appealing to other aspects of doctors' practices that are important to them, such as professional ethics, and competence and qualifications; that is, being a good doctor both morally and technically.

Remuneration of general practitioners has attracted much interest among health economists. We believe that the theoretical attention of SID is out of proportion for its relevance. When fee for service is deliberatively intended to increase service provision, we would expect physicians to respond by recommending that patients use more of their services. Hence, demand would be induced. The question is whether it is being induced beyond the level that patients would prefer—if they had the same level of information as the doctor. We believe that professional codes of ethics would stop the vast majority of doctors allowing this to be the case.

In their role as gatekeepers, GPs hold a unique position in the health care system. The only way in which patients can get access to hospitals and specialist care in many countries is following referral from a GP. Hence, if GPs are permissive in making referrals, they put increased pressure on hospitals' resources. Much of the literature on GP remuneration has been concerned with efficiency in terms of value for money within primary care only. Activity-based remuneration systems appear to improve efficiency and are therefore preferred to salary systems in which doctors have no financial incentive to increase productivity. However, given the important role of GPs in the referral decisions and hence the cost consequences of their choices in secondary care, given also the use of pharmaceuticals and the costs of sick leave, we would argue that any evaluation of the efficiency of a remuneration system must focus on the wider resource impact outside the GP practice.

Suggested reading

Rice, T. (2006) The physician as the patient's agent. In *The Elgar Companion to Health Economics* (ed. A. Jones). Cheltenham: E. Elgar Publishing.

Iversen, T. and Lurås, H. (2006) Capitation and incentives in primary care. In *The Elgar Companion to Health Economics* (ed. A. Jones). Cheltenham: E. Elgar Publishing.

Léger, P. T. (2008) Physician payment mechanisms. In *Financing health care: New ideas for a changing society* (ed. M. Lu and E. Jonsson). Weinheim: Wiley-VCH Verlag.

Exercises

1. Why all these sophisticated remuneration systems for GPs? Are they lazy? Are they greedy? Why are they not just practising in accordance with their professional codes of ethics, independent of financial self-interest?

2. Give some examples of the international variation in blended GP remuneration systems.

3. Can we choose an optimal remuneration system for GPs without taking account of the way in which hospitals are being reimbursed? Explain why or why not.

Chapter 11

Secondary care: reimbursing hospitals

This chapter presents three alternative reimbursement systems for hospitals and discusses the pros and cons of each system. In their pure form, none of these systems emerges as the ideal solution, which explains why we observe blended systems in practice.

While to some extent the concepts used differ, there are clear parallels between the payment systems used in primary care and those used in secondary care. For hospitals, the alternative principles of the various reimbursement systems are classified along two key dimensions: *retrospective vs prospective* systems, and *fixed vs variable* systems (Jegers *et al.*, 2002). In fixed systems, the payment does not vary with activity; but it does in variable systems. In retrospective systems providers' own cost are fully reimbursed ex post, while in prospective systems payments are determined ex ante without any link to the real costs incurred by the individual provider. See Table 11.1.

The first combination—*fixed and retrospective*—simply does not make sense. It would be like the payer handing over a lump sum to each hospital at the end of the year independently of the hospital's activity level during the year. The second combination—*fixed and prospective*—has been much used in tax-financed public systems in which hospitals receive a set budget that is normally based on their previous year's budget and activity, as well as the planned activity for the coming year. The third combination—*variable and retrospective*—has been used in private as well as public insurance systems. After patients are treated and costs have been incurred, hospitals simply bill the third-party payer.

Table 11.1 A typology for hospital payment systems

	Retrospective	*Prospective*
Fixed	Not applicable	Annual global budgets
Variable	Fee for service	Per patient/case

The fourth combination—*variable and prospective*—refers to when hospitals are reimbursed according to their *activity* (number of patients treated, normally adjusted for types of diagnosis), but not according to their actual *costs* incurred. This alternative is also referred to as activity-based financing (ABF), although, by definition, the retrospective variable alternative is an activity-based financing system as well. To add to the possible confusion, this alternative is also referred to as a prospective payment system (PPS), although—again by definition—the fixed prospective alternative is a prospective payment system as well. Whatever the label or acronym, the *variable prospective* combination is a relatively new provider payment system that can be observed in many countries when health care reforms are being implemented.

When assessing the value of each of the three possible combinations, we need to ask: what should the reimbursement system achieve or contribute towards? The preferred system should ideally achieve three things simultaneously: i) cost efficiency, i.e. produce each service (with a specified quality) in the cheapest possible way; ii) allocative efficiency, i.e. produce the right combination of health services (in accordance with health care priorities); and iii) cost containment (budget discipline). Unfortunately, in their pure form none of the three reimbursement systems would simultaneously achieve all three objectives. A crucial issue in the discussion about incentives for efficiency and budget discipline is: who carries the financial risk—the third-party payer or the provider?

11.1 **Retrospective variable: cost reimbursement**

Retrospective per diem pricing used to be a common reimbursement system in many countries. In publicly funded national health services one would divide the hospital's total costs in the previous year by the number of patient days. This per diem price would then be adjusted for inflation and multiplied by the number of patients treated in the following year—which would then determine the scale of the hospital's reimbursement.

In private health insurance systems the retrospective reimbursement system was even simpler: register all costs incurred in the treatment of each individual patient and send the bill to the insurance company, which would then reimburse the hospital.

Such retrospective reimbursement systems have inbuilt incentives to increase length of stay, to provide more diagnostic tests, and to increase quality—all of which escalate cost. When all the costs incurred are to be reimbursed, the hospital does not face any financial risks related to paying for all the resources used in the treatments it provides. Because of these cost inefficiencies and lack of budget discipline, it is no wonder that third-party payers started looking for alternative ways in which to reimburse providers.

11.2 **Prospective fixed budgets**

One simple solution to lack of budget discipline is for the third-party payer to allocate fixed annual budgets to providers, something which happened in Norway in 1980. This simple remedy was also used in many other countries with publicly funded national health services, e.g. the UK's NHS until recently.

Prospective fixed budgets mean that the third-party payer avoids all financial risk; it is the provider who faces the risk. If hospitals admit too many patients and/or provide too many services, they end up with a financial deficit. If they adhere to the financial constraint and there is excess demand for their services, either directly from patients or indirectly through referral of patients from GPs, the consequences are waiting lists and dissatisfied patients. When hospitals refuse to accept full responsibility for these two undesirable alternatives (deficits or waiting lists), a political 'blame-game' arises: hospitals blame politicians for allocating inadequate budgets, while politicians blame hospitals for being inefficient.

Hospitals are more likely to win at least some of this blame game, in the sense that politicians will allocate additional budgets towards the end of the budget period. The political cost of blaming hospitals by giving them sole responsibility is simply too high. Thus the system of prospective fixed budgets evaporates: we observe a shift from what are intended to be 'hard' budgets to 'soft' budgets. When hospitals know that they will be allocated additional funding—since the political costs for not doing so are too high—they have less incentive for being cost efficient.

However, this reimbursement alternative with fixed budgets for each provider does not apply in private insurance systems, in which patients have a legal contract with the third-party payer (insurance company) that guarantees their entitlement to treatments.

11.3 **Prospective variable**

This alternative emerges as the solution to different problems in different institutional settings. In the USA, the federal government introduced the Medicare

Prospective Payment System (PPS) in 1983 as a way to change hospital behaviour through financial incentives that encourage more cost-efficient management. In the tax-financed Norwegian health service, a similar prospective system was introduced in 1997 as the means of increasing the number of elective treatments, in order to fulfil the waiting list guarantee adopted by parliament. Increased funding within the existing system of block grants to the county councils was expected to result in financial leakages to other sectors for which the counties were responsible. More recently, variable prospective payment systems have been introduced in other countries, e.g. known as 'payment by result' (PBR) in the UK. Furthermore, in private health insurance settings, hospital reimbursement is increasingly based on prospectively estimated costs rather than retrospectively incurred costs.

Typically, the prospective variable system is based on a classification of all hospital admissions according to the homogeneity of the resource use and clinical characteristics (principal and secondary diagnoses, procedure, age). The most commonly used classification system is called *diagnosis-related group* (DRG). For each DRG, a national average cost is estimated that forms the basis for the national tariff of DRG cost weights, on which hospitals fees are determined, i.e. the fee varies with the diagnosis and required treatment category for each patient. This tariff is then used for all providers independently of any local cost variations that reflect differences in hospital efficiency.

Note the three separate facets of the DRG system: First, it is a diagnosis *classification* system, based on the homogeneity of the resource use and clinical characteristics. Second, it is a cost *information* system, based on national average costs in the average hospital. Third, it is a *reimbursement* system: up to 100% of the average treatment costs of the DRG to which the admitted patient belongs.

Compared with fee for service, the experience with DRG-based reimbursement is that cost efficiency improves. Compared with total budgets, the Norwegian experience is that technical efficiency in terms of DRG points increases; but the effect is less uniform with respect to cost efficiency (Biørn *et al.*, 2003). The effect on cost efficiency depends on how input prices are affected: if the transition from fixed budgets is accompanied by greater use of paid overtime (since operating theatres are used for longer hours), the effect may well be negative. Input prices may also increase if hospitals face 'soft' budget constraints so that inefficient hospitals can acquire more input factors. And last, if better performance one year implies tougher performance standards the following year, there is a 'ratchet effect' that reduces the incentive to improve efficiency, since the payer will claim the increased revenue that the provider is generating (Hagen and Kaarbøe, 2006).

In general, if input prices are unaffected, there is reason to believe that case-based reimbursement will improve cost efficiency. However, cost containment may be negatively affected, when hospitals have no financial constraints to stop increasing admissions. A known concern is the incentive for patient selection and dumping, i.e. hospitals select the 'easy cases' that require less than average resources, and dump 'heavy cases' whose treatment will incur costs beyond the fees in the DRG tariff. Furthermore, there is the problem of 'DRG creep', i.e. the incentive to classify admissions in a way that maximizes reimbursement by adding secondary diagnoses which generate higher fees.

11.4 **Macro vs micro level**

In countries with tax-financed health care, it appears that the major concern among policy makers about the effects of the variable prospective reimbursement model is the lack of cost control at the macro level. A suggested solution is to combine a fixed-budget model at the macro level with an activity-based model at the micro level. Under such a regime, parliament could decide the total national health care budget and allocate it across regions or health districts on a capitation basis (eventually needs-adjusted depending on age and social class). At the sub-national level the intermediary fundholder would then reimburse the providers according to their activity.

This combined model appears to be a very attractive one for purchasers, in that they face no financial risk, while simultaneously they can exercise some control over providers through the inbuilt efficiency incentive. However, since the purchaser's available budget is fixed and the total production of DRG points is unknown at the start of the period, the reimbursed fee per DRG point will be decided at the end of the period—*after* hospitals have reported their production of DRG points. Of course, the model is less attractive for the hospitals, which carry all financial risks. Since the DRG prices that determine their revenues are not given, this is like producing and selling goods with unknown prices!

11.5 **Conclusion**

Unfortunately, *none* of the three hospital reimbursement models is consistent with all three policy objectives of cost efficiency, allocative efficiency, *and* cost containment. Table 11.2 summarizes the behavioural response and the pros and cons of the models.

The behavioural response to *variable retrospective* reimbursement is to increase the provision of services to each patient admitted. The resulting over-provision of services implies cost escalation and cost inefficiency. Allocative

Table 11.2 Three reimbursement models and their respective effects

	Retrospective variable (fee for service)	Prospective fixed (global budgets)	Prospective variable (activity based)
Behavioural response	*Increase* provision of services to each patient admitted	Waiting lists	*Reduce* provision of services to each patient admitted
Cost containment	Very bad	Very good	Bad
Cost efficiency	Very bad	?	Very good
Allocative efficiency	Good	Good	?

efficiency might be positive due to the fact that when all incurred costs are being reimbursed, there is no financial incentive to deviate from any politically determined priority criterion. In theory, though, it is difficult to envisage that a cost-*in*efficient system can be allocative efficient (see Chapter 2). Thus it might be more precise to say that the *degree* of waste is the same across all (groups of) patients treated.

The merit of the *fixed prospective* model is clearly cost containment. As to allocative efficiency, there is nothing in theory to suggest that global budgets will make hospitals avoid prioritized patient groups: the budget is fixed no matter which patients are being treated. As to the degree of waste, this appears to be somewhat more contentious. If the objective were plainly to maximize health, or the production of health care, hospitals would have an incentive to be cost efficient. However, all organizations prefer *some* slack, the optimal level of which is restricted by the simple connection: more slack → lower productivity → less income. Under a fixed-budget regime, however, there are no such links between income and slack, which suggests higher levels of slack. The behavioural response to fixed budgets is to put patients on the waiting list.

The behavioural response to *variable prospective* reimbursements is to admit patients but be restrictive with service provision. The merit of the system is primarily improved cost efficiency, while its shortcoming is the lack of cost control. As to allocative efficiency, different effects are seen at patient group level compared with at individual patient level. As long as fees reflect average costs, there is nothing in theory to suggest that prioritized patient groups are any less 'profitable' than other patient groups. However, at the individual patient level, there is an incentive to dump expensive patients. The extent to which this is done in practice will of course depend on regulations and ethical standards.

In conclusion, it seems quite clear that prospective payment systems are better than the retrospective alternative. The question is over fixed and/or variable, i.e. should we opt for a blended prospective system rather than either of the pure alternatives? If blended, the next question is which percentage of the average costs should be activity based? Clearly, there is no universally right or wrong answer. The Norwegian experience is one in which this has varied between 30% and 60%. Rather than reflecting new evidence for an optimal split, the percentage changes from one budget year to the next are the result of political compromises in parliament.

Finally, the search for the best reimbursement system in *secondary* care cannot be undertaken in isolation from which system exists in *primary* care. When patients are being referred from primary care physicians to hospitals, and then discharged to tertiary care or other types of follow-up outside hospitals, we need to broaden our analyses and look at integrated systems.

Suggested reading

Jegers, M., Kesteloot, K., De Graeve, D. and Gilles, W. (2002) A typology for provider payment systems in health care. *Health Policy*, 60 (3):255–73.

McKee, M. and Healy, J. (ed.) (2002) Ho*spitals in a Changing Europe*. Buckingham: Open University Press (available at http://www.euro.who.int/observatory).

Magnussen, J., Hagen, T. P. and Kaarbø, O. (2007) Centralized or decentralized? A case study of Norwegian hospital reform. *Social Science and Medicine*, 64, 2129–37.

Exercises

1. Why is it so difficult for policy makers to stick to 'hard' budgets for hospitals?

2. Give some examples of the international variation in hospital reimbursement systems.

3. Discuss some potential negative consequences that an activity-based prospective payment system may have on attitudes and behaviour of health care personnel.

Chapter 12

Integrating the health care provider system

This chapter moves from the partial effects of alternative reimbursement systems within primary and secondary care to considering the links *between* provider levels. Particular emphasis is put on how GPs' decisions have cost implications in other parts of the health care system.

If each provider level were operating in a vacuum, in the sense that its decisions had no cost implications for health care providers at other levels, then of course partial analyses are justified. However, a characteristic feature of the health sector is that most of its 'customers' flow through at least two provider levels. Before discussing key parts of the health care provider system and the various ways in which the parts might be integrated, we will make a brief overview of some recent policy reforms in the payment of primary and secondary care providers.

12.1 Combinations of payment systems in primary and secondary care

In what follows, the focus will be on how some alternative *combinations* of provider payments in primary and secondary care seem to have evolved over the last 50 years. The policy context is set in a rich country with publicly funded health care, such as Norway or the UK.

When health care expenditures took a smaller slice of the total public budget, the fiscal issue of cost containment was not too much of a policy concern. Retrospective variable payment systems were used, fee for service in primary care and per diem rates in secondary care.

For reasons explained in the previous chapter, health care costs gradually increased. Since total costs in specialist care were much higher than in primary care, hospitals became the target for cost-containment interventions. Furthermore, when hospitals were publicly owned, it was politically more feasible to regulate this part of the health sector than primary care, which traditionally has been run by independent practitioners (physicians, physiotherapists) in small private practices. GPs have always had a much stronger autonomy and self-governing status, and have therefore been more difficult to regulate than hospitals. Thus, prospective fixed budgets for hospitals appeared to be the best remedy for solving the problem of health care cost escalation.

When budgets become fixed independent of activity, hospitals no longer have the incentive to increase admissions. The most immediate consequence is hospital waiting lists, something that carries a heavy political burden. As a result of a 'blame game' between politicians and hospital managers, what are intended as 'hard' budgets turn to 'soft' budgets in exchange for a promise to reduce waiting lists.

One important positive effect of this change from *retrospective variable* to *prospective fixed* hospital financing is the incentive for improved cost efficiency. A crucial part of hospital managers' increased cost consciousness is to control the most important cost item, namely salaries. However, if hospital clinicians' wages do not keep pace with those of their colleagues in primary care, it is necessary to curb GPs' incomes as well. A change from fee for service to capitation improves cost control (see Table 10.1), and may hence be an effective way of stopping a potential flow of doctors from hospitals to primary care. Furthermore, a capitation system will regulate the labour market for primary care providers much more effectively than fee for service.

This change from fee for service to capitation has some positive effects: less supplier-induced demand and better cost control—but only *within* primary care. While fee for service has a do-it-yourself incentive, capitation has the reverse: *do not* do it yourself, but refer patients to specialists.

The combination of capitation in primary care and fixed budgets in secondary care is fine for cost containment. The big problem lies in the excess demand for secondary care—as manifested in hospital waiting lists. Gatekeepers in primary care have abdicated, sending flows of patients to the closed hospital gates. The consequence is excess demand. One way to open these gates was to offer a financial incentive through prospective activity-based financing.

There is no simple single explanation for the increased health care spending observed in most rich countries over the last decades. Still, *one* explanation might be the aggregate incentive effects in the popular reforms that have been implemented for paying primary and secondary care providers. The combination of capitation in primary care and prospective activity-based financing in second-ary care appears to be a nightmare for national treasuries! GPs have an incentive to increase referrals, and hospitals have an incentive to admit the increased flow of patients.

Prior to the reforms towards more activity-based financing of hospitals, there was in some countries an era of 'internal markets' as a solution to some big health sector problems: inefficiencies in hospital care, long waiting lists, and cost escalations. The idea was that the *flow of patients* from primary care to secondary care should be accompanied by a *flow of money* to cover the costs of further treatment, i.e. when GPs make referrals they should be confronted with the resource implications of their decisions. In the jargon of politicians, 'the money should follow the patient'. Before discussing various incentives and policies aiming to improve GPs' cost consciousness, let us illustrate the crucial role of GPs within the 'body' of the health care provider system.

12.2 The 'body' of the health care provider system

Through their referral decisions and clinical practice, general practitioners make claims on how much resource other parts of the health care system should put up for the treatment of their patients. Except for acute and emergency care, in many countries patients need to see a GP before they can obtain access to specialist care. Furthermore, patients need prescription from a GP to get their medication, and people usually need to see a doctor to be eligible for sickness benefit.

Health care provider systems vary between countries, depending on the ways in which they are financed and the extent of public regulations. But a key distinction is that between *primary care* and *specialist (or secondary) care*. The precise line between the two levels is blurred, though, reflecting that some services provided by GPs in one country are provided by hospitals in another. Rather than classifying the two levels according to which services they provide, it might be more useful to consider the specialist care level as one that nor-mally requires referral from a general practitioner, or at least is subsequent to having been seen by a GP.

In some countries there exists an intermediate level, anything from the con-cept of a large-scale polyclinic in an urban area (a collaboration of many GPs, offering a wider set of services), to a small-scale district hospital in a rural area. In some settings, the concept of specialist care refers to specialist hospitals, e.g. heart clinics. However, in the current context, specialist care refers to general—as well as specialist—hospitals, and even independent specialists, as long as patients have been referred from a GP or have been admitted for reasons of acute or emergency treatment.

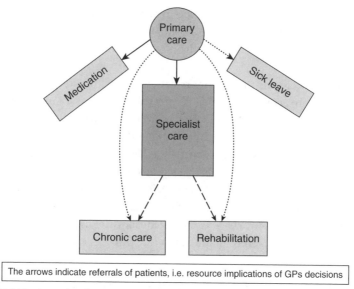

Fig. 12.1 The key role of GPs within the 'body' of the health care provider system.

Beyond the secondary care level, there is a provider level to which discharged patients may be referred, often called *tertiary care*. In principle, this can be separated into two different branches depending on the patient's prognosis: chronic care or rehabilitation. If further health improvements are likely, follow-up rehabilitation is an option. If *no* further health improvements are likely, chronic care is offered to the terminally ill, or nursing homes are available for the elderly. In many countries, there has been much interest in integrated care or the continuing care interface, e.g. more nursing home beds will reduce the need for more hospital beds.

These parts form the *'body' of the health care provider system*, as illustrated in Figure 12.1. Primary care is represented by the head; specialized care forms the trunk; medication and sick leave are the hands; and chronic care and rehabilitation are the feet. The arrows from the head indicate referrals and hence claims for resources provided by the other parts of the health care body. The solid arrows indicate that referrals from GPs are most likely to be required, while dotted arrows indicate that GPs may have an important influence in determining the amount of resources provided by the other parts.

The relative sizes of the resource provided by the different parts will of course vary, depending on what the country can afford, how the health care system is organized, and how generous the social insurance system is regarding eligibilities for sickness benefit. In Norway, the relative sizes of the parts in expenditure terms are: prescribed medication costs 1.5 times that of primary care

(GP practices); specialized care costs 10 times that of primary care; the total cost of chronic care and rehabilitation is 5 times that of primary care; and sick leave costs are 15–20 times that of primary care. While the relative sizes of the different parts vary between countries, one crucial lesson is that the costs *inside* primary care are tiny compared with the total costs that decisions within primary care generate *outside*. Hence, the policy concern for the gatekeeping role of GPs.

When designing policy interventions, it is important to acknowledge the *dual agent* role that GPs play: i) as agent for the patient (see Chapter 3), including the crucial decisions on referring the patient to services offered by other parts of the provider system, and ii) as agent for society, recognizing that the opportunity costs of these other services must be taken into account (i.e. the benefits that will be forgone by other patients).

12.3 Interventions: integration and incentives

Since GPs face no costs when referring their patients to hospitals, nor when prescribing medication or when acceding to a patient's request for a sick note, they have no financial incentives to modify their demand for such services. There are principally two different ways in which GPs can be forced to take these cost implications into account: financial incentives or regulatory restrictions in their freedom to request resources from other parts of the health care provider system.

12.3.1 Financial carrots and sticks: internal markets

To economists, the most intuitive solution lies with the idea of 'internal markets'. Remember, 'there is no such thing as free health care', so the argument goes that services should be priced in accordance with marginal costs, and allocated to those patients whose needs GPs consider sufficiently high to justify the costs of the services. By becoming budget holders, GPs purchase services, that carry costs, rather than make referrals for services that are *seemingly* free. In general, when decision makers are faced with the costs of their choices, they will modify their demands—consistent with the simple logic of the demand curve.

The idea of internal markets for specialist health care is fine in theory, but quite difficult when put into practice. There are problematic issues related to transaction costs, uncertainty, cream-skimming, etc. In theory, drug budgets are easier, since they involve less transaction cost (price lists of drugs can easily be made available) and less uncertainty on the cost consequences. Analogous to internal markets for specialist care, a GP can be equipped with a separate budget that specifies how much total medication he can prescribe to all patients on his list. However, he does not need the budget to be transferred to his practice.

An alternative is for the third-party payer to issue expenditure caps on pharmaceutical prescriptions—a policy applied in Germany.

As with the internal markets for specialist care, the incentive for the GP is to choose the most cost-effective drugs: instead of opting for costly new drugs, they will be more inclined to prescribe the cheaper generic alternatives. Opposition to cost-containment measures of this kind can be understood if you recall the 'revenue—expenditure—income' identity in Part 3: expenditure caps imply *income caps* for those who sell medication. A popular policy for the third-party payer, then, is unpopular for those who receive their income from the capped expenditures.

The use of prices can be implemented between any two parts of the health care provider system in which one part's decisions have implications for the other part's costs. In some countries, there are pseudo-markets between specialist care and chronic care, intended to make nursing homes admit elderly patients who are stuck in the corridors of hospitals after cure. The policy is one in which a specialized hospital can charge a fee to the local nursing home for each additional night in hospital after the patient is considered ready to be discharged to a nursing home.

The urge to implement internal prices between different health care provider levels is particularly relevant if there are different third-party payers behind each level. Although all provider levels in some countries are publicly financed, there might well be an intricate institutional system whereby one government agency has the financial responsibility for one part, while another agency has the responsibility for another part. In Norway, for instance, a specific government body reimburses prescribed medication, the ministry of health is the third-party payer for specialist care, municipalities have the financial responsibility for chronic care and some primary care, and sickness benefits are paid from a different part of the public purse. No wonder immense public administration challenges are involved in making each provider level take into account the resource implications of their isolated decisions beyond their own budgets.

The rationale behind internal markets is to make decision makers become concerned with cost consequences in other provider levels. An alternative is to develop guidelines that restrict the clinical freedom to request the use of less effective resources. A further alternative is to introduce 'targets', although in practical health policy targets relate more to quality and performance.

12.3.2 **Guidelines and targets**

Clinical guidelines—covering which medical procedures a clinician could or should choose in different diagnostic cases—serve two principal purposes: to ensure expected quality of outcomes, and to avoid cost-ineffective procedures. In the current context, we are primarily concerned with the latter, i.e. how to limit clinicians' freedom to demand all sorts of health care resources on behalf of their patient.

Although total costs of pharmaceuticals are only about 10–15% of total health care expenditures in most countries, it is interesting to note how health policy focuses on restricting the prescription of cost-inefficient pharmaceuticals, compared with policies to restrict GPs' referrals to unnecessary specialist care, or policies directed at restricting patients' requests for sick leave.

In addition to the use of guidelines and regulations, there certainly are other ways in which to curb the cost consequences of GPs' decisions in other parts of the health care system. One is vertical organizational integration, in which GPs are employed by the hospital; another is the creation of HMOs (health maintenance organizations), which include primary and specialized care—and even tertiary care. A looser form of collaboration is to establish 'practice coordinators' in a dialogue between GPs and hospital clinicians.

More recently there has been an increased use of 'payment for performance', whereby a financial premium is linked to achievements on a set of 'quality indicators' or 'targets'. Such types of incentives have been tried out in primary care as well as in hospitals. Interestingly, the focus of such policies appears to be more about improving quality of service provision and health outcomes than about cost consciousness. In principle, however, 'targets' as a management tool may also include 'cost-consciousness indicators'.

12.4 **Conclusion**

Remember the conclusion from the previous two chapters: that no single payment system—whether in primary care or specialized care—emerges as the ideal one. It should come as no surprise therefore that things are even more complicated when considering alternative *combinations* of payment systems for each provider level. Since decisions to opt for unnecessary sick leave very much depend on how generous sickness benefits are, as well as patients' preferences for income vs leisure, we will set to one side that part of health-related costs. We will also set aside the question of equity by assuming there is 'equal access for equal need'; and we will assume that there are no problems of allocative efficiency. What remain are the two principal issues of cost efficiency and overall cost containment in the aggregated health care provider system.

The simplest way to achieve the objective of cost containment in the system is to divide the total health sector budget between each provider. When making referrals, GPs would just have to hope that medication and specialized care will be available for their patients. However, the result of this approach is waiting lists for specialized care and 'soft' budgeting for medication. Furthermore, there is little incentive for cost efficiency in this payment system.

The idea behind the GP budget-holding model is very appealing: it implies cost containment, and it has an inbuilt cost-efficiency incentive. Cost containment is achieved when the third-party payer decides first of all how much in total to spend on GP services, prescribed medication, and referrals to specialist care, and then divides this aggregate budget between independent GP fund holders. GPs then have the incentive in their clinical practice to be cost conscious in their demand for medication and specialist care for their patients—provided of course that the GP aims to do as much good as possible to their patients' health, given the available budget. Unfortunately, the model has proven to be difficult when put into practice.

A final word of caution is the danger that the increased emphasis on financial incentives and internal markets between provider levels may affect the attitudes and focus of clinicians. Instead of considering health care personnel in other provider levels as their professional colleagues, they are seen as business people with whom to negotiate. Participation in professional dialogue over what is considered a sound, sober, and sensible clinical practice might well prove to be more effective than the use of financial carrots and sticks.

Suggested reading

Enthoven, A. C. (1991) Internal market reform of the British National Health Service. *Health Affairs*, 10 (3): 60–70.

Saltman, R., Bankauskaite, V. and Vrangbæk, K. (2005) *Decentralization in health care—strategies and outcomes. Buckingham: Open University Press (available at* http://www.euro.who.int/observatory).

Bevan, G. and Hood, C. (2006) What's measured is what matters: Targets and gaming in the English public health care system. *Public Administration*, 84 (3): 517–38.

Exercises

1. What are the relative sizes in expenditure terms of the different parts of 'the health care provider body' (Figure 12.1) in your country?

2. Find examples of 'internal markets' between health care provider levels in your country.

3. Discuss how the different health care provider levels may collaborate—without the use of financial incentives—in attempting to improve overall cost containment.

Part 5

Economic evaluation and priority setting

The most important issue when deciding whether to provide a new health care programme is the extent to which it improves health. The essence of medical research has always dealt with how new interventions improve patients' health. More recently this focus on documenting outcomes has gained increasing attention through new concepts and professional associations, such as 'evidence-based medicine' and the Cochrane collaboration.

While Archie Cochrane himself held that 'all effective care should be free', health care certainly does not come for free, inasmuch as it is not cost free. Nobel prize-winning economist Milton Friedman was fond of the old saying, 'There's no such thing as a free lunch,' meaning that there are costs involved in providing it—and these are paid by someone other than the person enjoying the lunch. Although patients can be provided with seemingly 'free' health care, society—through its third-party payer—is faced with the cost of producing it. Therefore, 'there is no such thing as free health care.' The more a particular health care programme costs, the fewer resources are available for other programmes. When we are concerned with the potential health improvements for *all* people, cost becomes the second most important issue in the evaluation of alternative health care programmes.

Here lies the heart of economic evaluation methodologies—in the comparison of costs with outcomes. An economic evaluation is a *systematic and explicit measurement, valuation, and comparison of costs and outcomes*. It takes a *societal perspective* in that it is concerned with the resource use of the whole society rather than merely the particular institution that provides the service. Further, it is concerned with the wider benefits to all members of society and not only the health effects in the treated patients. Figure 13.1 illustrates two key

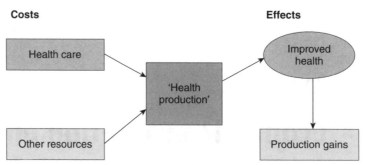

Fig. 13.1 Costs and effects/benefits.

types of costs and two key types of effects/benefits. The benefits stem from improved health per se and the productivity gains that are the *consequences* of improved health. This analytical distinction has a parallel in a seminal health economics model (Grossman, 1972), which distinguished between the consumption benefits from health care (the utility of being in improved health) and the investment benefits (the utility of the increased income that the improved health will generate).

Note also the distinction between *non-monetary* health improvements (in the ellipse) and monetary production gains. Hence, when comparing costs and effects, we cannot aggregate health effects with production gains. The latter will have to be subtracted from the costs, in order to compare net societal costs with health effects. An alternative solution is to value health effects in money terms.

The ways in which benefits are measured appears to be the distinguishing feature of the various economic evaluation techniques. Table 13.1 distinguishes the methods depending on whether benefits have been measured in monetary terms or not, and whether benefits are based on preferences or not. When benefits are measured in money, they by definition become comparable to costs. An economic evaluation in which benefits are measured in monetary terms is referred to as a cost—benefit analysis (CBA). However, economists tend to reserve the CBA label for those analyses that have their theoretical basis

Table 13.1 A taxonomy of economic evaluation techniques

		Benefits measured in money terms	
		Yes	*No*
Benefits based on preferences	*Yes*	CBA (welfare economics)	CEA (CUA)
	No	CBA	CEA

in neoclassical welfare economics. Here, benefits are based on preferences that reflect the consumers' valuations, e.g. as expressed through their willingness to pay. Although many economists might not use the label CBA when benefits are *not* based on preferences, non-economists might do so.

If benefits are *not* measured in monetary terms, some sort of cost-effectiveness analysis (CEA) is being used. An important class of CEA in the health economics literature is what has come to be labelled 'cost—utility analysis' (CUA). The use of 'utility' here is because the benefit is claimed to be some measure of individual utility from health.

In Table 13.1, the vertical distinction is clear-cut in that benefits are either measured in monetary terms or they are not. The horizontal distinction separates out those techniques that do not have *any* bases in preferences. Among those techniques that do attempt to measure preferences, there is a wide range of possible sources of value, from those evaluations that make only very rough estimates of the utility from a health state to those that proclaim that preferences over all attributes of a programme have been assessed.

Nevertheless, whichever economic evaluation label is used, when comparing a new treatment with an existing one, we start with two simple ordinal questions: i) is the new programme more or less *effective*? and ii) is it more or less *costly*? Figure 13.2. illustrates what has come to be termed 'the cost-effectiveness plane' with its four alternative combinations. If the new programme turns out to be less effective and more costly, forget it! If the new programme is more

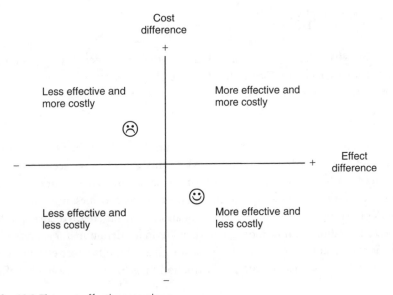

Fig. 13.2 The cost-effectiveness plane.

effective and less costly, implement it. If the new programme is more effective *and* more costly, or if it is less effective but less costly, we would need to proceed from these two simple ordinal questions to a more rigorous economic evaluation.

For now we will consider the most general representation of what the various economic evaluation techniques have in common: namely, the comparison of costs and benefits. A programme evaluation starts out by *identifying* and *quantifying* (in physical units) the items in question and categorizes them into being benefit items, indexed by i (B_i) or cost items, indexed by j (C_j). Costs are *valued* in monetary terms, (V_j). Benefits can be *valued* in three different ways (V_i): in monetary terms, in non-monetary terms such as quality-of-life indices, or in physical or natural units, i.e. 'in themselves', such as lives saved. Since benefits and costs occur at different points in time (t), a discount rate, r, is used to adjust for such time differences.

The policy question to which an economic evaluation is intended to provide an answer is whether the programme is worth pursuing. In economic terms, this is essentially the *potential Pareto criterion*, which looks at whether the gainers can potentially compensate the losers, i.e. is the value to the beneficiaries larger than the losses to those who bear the costs? And, in cost—benefit terms, is the present value of the future stream of benefits greater than the future stream of costs? Using the symbols suggested above, this net present value (NPV) can be specified as in Equation 13.1:

$$\text{NPV} = \frac{\Sigma_t \Sigma_i (V_{it}{}^* B_{it})}{\Sigma_t (1+r)^t} - \frac{\Sigma_t \Sigma_j (V_{jt}{}^* C_{jt})}{\Sigma_t (1+r)^t} \tag{13.1}$$

If this NPV calculation is greater than zero, then implement the programme; if it is not, then do not. Clearly, for this general formula to make sense, the first term must be measured in the same unit as the second, i.e. benefits must be valued in monetary terms. Hence, Equation 13.1 refers—by definition—to CBA (see Table 13.1).

However, just as apples and oranges cannot be added together, nor can apples be *subtracted* from oranges (or vice versa). So when we decide to value benefits in health terms, the first term of Equation 13.1 is expressed in a different unit from the second term, and the formula becomes meaningless. In order to compare costs and benefits, Equation 13.1 is therefore rearranged to become a ratio. The non-monetarized benefits in the denominator are referred to as *effects*, and so Equation 13.2 is the formula behind the cost-effectiveness ratio (CER). Consistent with the distinction in Table 13.1 between benefits and effects, we change the index from B to E when we refer to units of non-monetary health effects:

$$\text{CER} = \frac{\dfrac{\Sigma_t \Sigma_j (V_{jt}{}^* C_{jt})}{\Sigma_t (1+r)^t}}{\dfrac{\Sigma_t \Sigma_i (V_{it}{}^* E_{it})}{\Sigma_t (1+r)^t}} \tag{13.2}$$

This ratio does not in itself offer any policy-relevant information. It is only when compared with the ratios from alternative programmes that a new programme's relative value can be assessed.

Health care decision makers are often faced with the comparison between a *new* treatment programme and an existing one. What matters then is the *incremental costs* of the new and the existing, compared with their *incremental effects*. Below, the existing treatment is referred to as the *comparator*, which is supposed to reflect current best practice. This is to answer the question: can the incremental costs be justified by the incremental effects? The incremental cost-effectiveness ratio (ICER) in Equation 13.3 follows from Equation 13.2 and expresses the ratio between the incremental costs and the incremental effects:

$$\text{ICER} = \frac{\dfrac{\Sigma_t \Sigma_j (V_{jt}{}^* C_{jt})_{NEW}}{\Sigma_t (1+r)^t} - \dfrac{\Sigma_t \Sigma_j (V_{jt}{}^* C_{jt})_{COMP}}{\Sigma_t (1+r)^t}}{\dfrac{\Sigma_t \Sigma_i (V_{it}{}^* E_{it})_{NEW}}{\Sigma_t (1+r)^t} - \dfrac{\Sigma_t \Sigma_i (V_{it}{}^* E_{it})_{COMP}}{\Sigma_t (1+r)^t}} \tag{13.3}$$

The core of the ICER can be simplified as in Equation 13.3a, which denotes the incremental present value of the *costs* of the new programme, C_{NEW}, and that of the comparator, C_{COMP} in the numerator, over the incremental present value of the *effects* of the new programme E_{NEW} and that of the comparator E_{COMP} in the denominator:

$$\text{ICER} = \frac{C_{NEW} - C_{COMP}}{E_{NEW} - E_{COMP}} = \frac{\Delta C}{\Delta E} \tag{13.3a}$$

The importance of the cost effectiveness of the comparator can be seen by looking at the simple algebra of Equation 13.3.a: the higher the cost of the comparator C_{COMP}, the more can be subtracted in the numerator; and/or the lower the effectiveness E_{COMP}, the less is being subtracted in the denominator. Hence, by choosing a cost-*in*effective comparator, a favourable ICER can easily be manipulated. Guidelines would normally dictate the basis for which the comparator is chosen: 'current best practice' or the most cost-effective alternative.

The remainder of this part of the book deals with the parameters in the above formulae. The next chapter deals with measuring and valuing *non-monetary* health effects (E), as well as methods for valuing *monetary* benefits (B). Chapter 14 discusses key principles in the estimation of costs (C) and the issue of time adjustments or discounting (r). Finally, Chapter 15 goes beyond the CBA and ICER formulae and discusses equity parameters that are not included in an economic evaluation, but nevertheless are considered relevant to setting priorities.

A characteristic feature of economic evaluations in practice is that of uncertainty in the estimation of key parameters. Data on health outcomes are normally based on trials with short study periods, implying that long-term effects beyond the length of the study period will have to be extrapolated using sophisticated modelling. Future cost figures are uncertain due to changes in technology and prices. If you want to learn about these methodological and modelling issues, and about new concepts such as cost-effectiveness—acceptability curves, you should consult other books, e.g. the standard reference, Drummond *et al.* (2005).

Recommended reading

Drummond, M. F., Sculpher, M. J., Torrance, G. W., O'Brien, B. J. and Stoddart, G. L. (2005) *Methods for the Economic Evaluation of Health Care Programmes.* Oxford: Oxford University Press.

Fox-Rushby, J. and Cairns, J. (2005) *Economic Evaluation.* Maidenhead: Open University Press.

Sorenson, C., Drummond, M. F. and Kanavos, P. (2008) Ensuring value for money in health care: The role of health technology assessment in the European Union. Available at http://www.euro.who.int/observatory

See also website, Pharmacoeconomic guidelines around the world: http://www.ispor.org/PEguidelines/index.asp

Chapter 13

Non-monetary effects and monetary benefits

This chapter deals with how to measure and value different degrees of health improvements—in health terms and in monetary terms. Beyond the valuation of improved health per se, the chapter discusses how to value the production gains following people's return to work as a possible *consequence* of the improved health.

The long history of medical research has used a wide range of outcome measures. Most of them are certainly useful and sensible for the specific purpose of inquiring into the extent to which new technologies do good, and whether a new procedure is any better than the existing one for the treatment of a specific disease. The discussion below focuses on how useful the various types of outcome measure are for the purpose of aiding resource-allocation decisions across different disease areas, e.g. should we treat cholera or other diseases, should we treat the physically disabled or the blind?

In the introductory chapter it was stated that any meaningful metric of health would have to include both quality and quantity. Looking back at Figure 1.1, we can interpret health care interventions as attempts at pushing the life span further out in the quality/quantity space: improve the health state and/or prolong the duration of life. Figure 13.3 illustrates gained health at the end of life, such as effects of preventative interventions. Curative interventions aim at improving health states earlier in life, the effects of which would have different durations.

The crucial issue is how to measure and value different types of health effects. The outline of this chapter is based on Table 13.1. We distinguish between

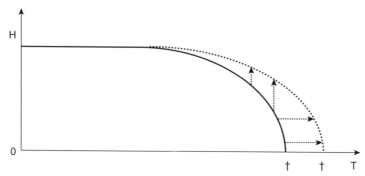

Fig. 13.3 Health gains at the end of life.

non-monetary health effects (E) that are relevant for cost-effectiveness analyses, and monetary benefits (B) that are used in cost—benefit analyses. However, some types of monetary benefits (production gains) are also relevant in the context of cost-effectiveness analyses. Additionally, we are concerned with the extent to which the outcome measure is *commensurable* or not.

An underlying message of this chapter is that *the QALY is a sophisticated measure of health* because it is a *commensurable preference-based* outcome measure. Everything is relative, so you need to learn about alternative types of measures, and what makes them *less* sophisticated in comparison.

13.1 **Incommensurable outcome measures**

Epidemiologists refer to 'end points' that can be 'intermediate', 'soft' or 'hard' depending on which types of events are being counted, and on how measurable different progression stages of a chronic disease might be. Which health effects are being identified, how are they measured, and how are they eventually valued?

Survival rates have been a widely used outcome measure in health. An intervention is counted a success if patients survive for, say, five years; it is counted a failure if they do not. This is obviously a very crude measure, since it does not distinguish between surviving one week or 4.9 years, or between surviving 5 years or 50 years. An alternative, therefore, is to count life years, so that the numeraire is no longer persons but years.

Death is the most final of all end points—and a 'hard' one in all senses. Lifetime data is seen as an objective indicator, which explains why increased lifetime is an attractive outcome measure. Since most clinical trials have a time horizon shorter than the time when all study participants have died, differences in survival rates have to be extrapolated, i.e. risk reductions are being translated into expected increased survival time. Survival rates and life years are commensurate terms for mortality, thus facilitating comparisons across programme areas. Still, they neglect any differences in morbidity.

Most types of events that are counted in clinical trials relate to morbidity. For chronic diseases that follow a detrimental progression, one would seek to identify specific diagnostic events. Cancer is characterized by the development of tumours. Screening programmes identify detected tumours and use differences in detection rates as an effect measure. However, detecting tumours says nothing about improved health, i.e. what the prospects are for *treating* cancer patients. For heart diseases, 'cardiovascular events' such as strokes or infarction are sought to be avoided, or perhaps more precisely, *postponed*. Hence, the effect of the intervention is measured as the extra time without a cardiovascular event. An even softer end point would be a specific blood-pressure level, i.e. the effect of the intervention is reduced blood pressure, something which is assumed to have a corresponding reduction in the risk of a cardiovascular event, implying gained time without that event.

In addition to identifying specific morbidity events, there are ways in which to describe differences in the levels of disease severity and hence measure the effects in terms of improvements along the chosen scale. A uni-dimensional scale is the simplest form, e.g. measure eyesight by the font size a person can read, or have a patient report their level of pain on a 10-point scale.

A more rigorous way is to identify several items or dimensions that are associated with the diagnosis or health condition being studied. There now exist more than 600 descriptive systems for health (www.proqolid.org), the vast majority of which are *condition or disease specific*. MADRS is a depression rating scale that includes 10 dimensions each described at seven levels. ODI (Oswestry disability index) is used for back pain patients, including 10 dimensions each described at six levels. By adding the level value of each dimension, you get an aggregate score that indicates the disease severity of the particular patient. A change in aggregate score value measures the effect of the intervention.

These two instruments are examples of widely used descriptive systems within each respective pathology. What is wrong with them? First, the effect scores from the instruments are incommensurable across disease areas, e.g. you cannot tell if a 12-point improvement on the MADRS instrument is any better than a 10-point improvement on the ODI instrument. Second, the instruments do not account for differences in duration. You cannot tell if a 20-point improvement that lasts for one year is as good as a 10-point change lasting for two years. Third, rarely are disease-specific instruments preference based. Hence, there is no valuation of the relative importance of each dimension for the people affected. Each dimension and each level change count the same, e.g. a given level change on 'suicidal thoughts' counts the same as on 'reduced sleep' when calculating a MADRS score. Furthermore, these scales have their focus on the dimension(s) of health that the given treatment *intends* to impact upon. 'Side effects' might sometimes be mentioned, but they are not measured such that they can be compared in a meaningful way with the positive effects.

These condition-specific outcome measures are inapplicable for aiding resource allocation in health care. For this purpose, an outcome measure should be able to: i) compare differences in improved mortality, i.e. the increased life expectancy or duration of time with improved health, ii) compare different types of improvements in morbidity, or health-related quality of life, across programme areas, iii) account for and compare improvements in *both* mortality and morbidity. Further, the valuation of the improvements should be based on the preferences of the affected parties. The *quality-adjusted life year* (QALY) was designed specifically to meet all these four requirements.

A somewhat intermediate class of outcome measure between the condition-specific instruments and the QALY are the so-called *health profiles* (such as WHOQOL and SF-36). These are generic descriptive systems for health and will therefore satisfy the second of the four requirements listed above. Since they do not satisfy the remaining three requirements, it is time to explain the QALY.

13.2 **Commensurable measures of health effects**

A leading proponent of the QALY, the late Alan Williams, referred to the QALY algorithm as a 'sophisticated measure of health'. Since QALYs are developed for the purpose of comparing health *gains*, let us concentrate on this stream of health. Other priority-relevant health streams such as the no-treatment profile and age will be discussed in Chapter 15.

13.2.1 **QALY: 'a sophisticated measure of health'**

For an individual, there are three possible types of future health gain; improved health-related quality of life, a longer lifetime, and an increased probability of survival. A usual simplification is to subsume the probability parameter and refer to *expected* remaining lifetime. The rationale for the QALY is to account for all of this into a common currency, along which all types—and combinations—of future health gains can be measured. Hence, through the application of this 'QALY currency', health gains become commensurable across programme areas.

Quality of life (Q) is usually measured on a scale of 0 to 1, where 1 refers to full health and 0 refers to death. Time (T) is counted in years. In short, QALYs are measured as the product of the average health-related quality of life (Q) and the lifetime (T) in that health. One year in full health therefore counts as one QALY. Consider now an intervention that improves longevity in full health by a given ΔT. The QALY gain (G) for this longer lifetime is then:

$$QALY_{G-T} = Q^* \Delta T \tag{13.4}$$

Alternatively, consider an intervention that improves the health state by ΔQ, but does not change the longevity. The QALY gain for this improved health-related quality of life is:

$$QALY_{G-Q} = \Delta Q^* T \tag{13.5}$$

It follows from Equations 13.4 and 13.5 that a programme that improves mortality becomes *commensurable* in health outcome terms with one that improves morbidity. Many interventions improve both quality *and* length of life. The shaded area in Figure 13.4 illustrates the QALY gain, where we have assumed that the health-related quality of life remains constant: without treatment, denoted as Q_0, and with treatment, denoted as Q_1. Time is accordingly denoted T_0 without treatment and T_1 with treatment.

The general formula for a QALY gain can be written as Equation 13.6, where the first term on the right-hand side refers to the expected health with treatment and the second term refers to the 'no-treatment profile'. The formula assumes only those two outcomes but can be extended for any number of mutually exclusive events.

$$QALY_G = Q_1^* T_1 - Q_0^* T_0 \tag{13.6}$$

This is all fine in theory, of course, but how in practice do we obtain reliable figures to put into this general—and very simple—formula?

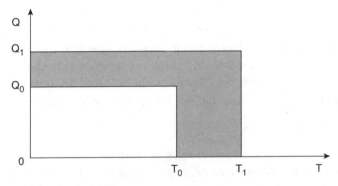

Fig. 13.4 Health gains in QALY terms.

Length of life with and without treatment is normally obtained from mortality tables and survival rates, while the probability of successful outcomes might be given by operation mortality rates. The measurement of T enables comparisons on an interval scale, e.g. the value of 10 years is twice as long as the value of 5 years (assuming there is no *discounting*, so that all years of life are given equal value, irrespective of when they occur—of which more in the next chapter). Similarly, we need quality of life to be measured on a scale with interval properties.

The challenge then is to use a descriptive system for health that is applicable across all types of morbidities, as well as being commensurable with mortality. There now exists a wide range of preference-based generic instruments (see Chapter 1). Their common feature is the attempt at describing physical, mental, and social well-being of people. They differ in how many items—or dimensions—of health are included, how the items are described, and how many levels each item can take. There is much disagreement in the literature on the pros and cons of the alternative instruments. When deciding which instrument to apply, many analysts may opt for a pragmatic solution and choose the one that is recommended in the economic evaluation guidelines. The EQ-5D instrument (www.euroqol.org) is the preferred one in the UK, according to the NICE guidelines.

Having decided which generic descriptive system to use, the next step is to decide how to measure and value the various combinations of health within the system. There are three main methods that have been used to value Q: visual analogue scale (VAS), standard gamble (SG) and time trade-off (TTO). The *visual analogue* (VAS) is a scale with fixed end points and equal intervals. It is usually illustrated vertically with a bottom value of 0, referred to as worst imaginable health (or dead), to a top value of 100, referred to as best imaginable (or full) health. The respondent is then asked to locate a given description of a health state on this scale.

The *standard gamble* (SG) presents a choice between being in a described health state for a given period of time, for certain, and a risk option with one better and one worse outcome (usually full health and death). Respondents are asked to specify the probability of a successful outcome that would make them indifferent to being in the described health as a certainty, or to choose the risk option. Formally, if Q_i is the value of the intermediate health state, p is the probability, Q_F is the value of full health and Q_D the value of death, then:

$$Q_i = p^*Q_F + (1 - p)Q_D \rightarrow Q_i = p \qquad (13.7)$$

The left-hand side is the value of being in the described health state and the right-hand side is the expected value of choosing the risk option. Hence, with $Q_F = 1$ and $Q_D = 0$, it follows that $Q_i = p$.

The *time trade-off* (TTO) represents a choice between a longer life in an inferior health state and a shorter life in full health. Usually, respondents are asked to imagine themselves in the described health state for a period of T years (e.g. $T = 10$), and then asked how many years they would be prepared to trade off in exchange for full health. Formally, if Q_i is the described state, and Q_F full health, t is the shorter time period in Q_F, and T is the given reference time, then:

$$Q_i^* T = t^* Q_F \rightarrow Q_i = t / T \tag{13.8}$$

The TTO reflects an explicit QALY choice, i.e. comparing quantity of life with quality of life. Figure 13.5 illustrates two equally good combinations of quantity and quality. Hence the two rectangles are equal in size, $(Q_i^* T = t^* Q_F)$: the shaded area one is willing to forgo is as big as the dotted one that is required as compensation.

In its simplest form, the TTO assumes constant proportional trade-off, meaning that the proportion of remaining lifetime one is willing to sacrifice is independent of how much time one has left. Studies suggest, however, that the less time an individual has left, the less they are prepared to sacrifice in order to improve the quality of life.

Many comparisons have been made of the health state values from these different approaches. VAS tends to give the lowest values and SG the highest, though not much higher than values from TTO. The theoretical reasons for these observed discrepancies appeal to intuitions. VAS differs from SG and TTO in that it does not involve a choice that requires the respondent to give up something. When no sacrifice is involved in giving a low value, it is easy to do so. With SG and TTO, a sacrifice *is* involved, either in terms of taking a risk of death (SG) or by giving up length of life (TTO). This would

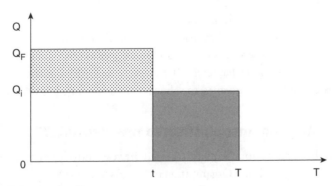

Fig. 13.5 Time trade-off.

restrict the individual's propensity to state a low implied value. The major difference between SG and TTO is that of certainty in TTO versus *un*certainty in SG, so risk-averse respondents would give higher implicit health state values under SG. Also, in the TTO, the fraction of time that the individual is asked to trade off is that which lies at the end of a given time, and so if these distant years are given less weight (i.e. if there is positive time preference), then respondents will give up these years more willingly.

In addition to these three methods for measuring an individual's value of Q, there is the person trade-off (PTO) method which looks at the *social value* (SV) of one health state compared with another (see Nord, 1995). It does this by asking respondents to think about a hypothetical choice between saving the life of one person and treating N persons in a described health state. The question is, how great would N have to be for the respondent to consider the two programmes equally good? The implicit social value of the described health state SV_i is then defined as:

$$SV_i = 1 - 1 / N \tag{13.9}$$

The values implied from the PTO are intended to reflect the social value of health states, as opposed to the individual utility that are implied from TTO and SG. Like the choice of descriptive system, there is much disagreement in the literature on which elicitation technique is the preferred one. Again, analysts may opt for those elicitation techniques that are accepted by national guidelines, which in the UK are TTO or SG.

The QALY has received much criticism in the literature. The relevance of this critique crucially depends on what a QALY should purport to be. If it is meant to reflect *individual utility* of health gains, there certainly are deficiencies in the ways in which parameter values are estimated. Empirical evidence shows that the assumptions of risk neutrality, and constant proportional trade-offs between Q and T, do not hold. If a QALY is meant to reflect *social value* of health care programmes, there certainly are other concerns people would include beyond differences in health gains. Empirical evidence shows that other streams of health matter, such as severity of illness and age, as well as other priority-relevant issues to be discussed in Chapter 15. If, however, the QALY is intended *only* to be a measure of health outcomes, the above criticism appears less relevant.

13.2.2 DALY: 'an unsophisticated inverted QALY'

DALY is the acronym for disability-adjusted life year, introduced by a research group in the World Health Organization in 1994. While QALYs were developed for the purpose of measuring health *gains*, DALYs were developed for the purpose of measuring the global burden of disease, i.e. the health *losses* associated with various causes of disease and injury. However, the DALY was also intended to be used as a metric for health effects in the denominator of cost-effectiveness ratios.

DALYs have important similarities with QALYs in the sense that they are metrics intended to be completely commensurable across mortalities and morbidities. Disability loss, D, is measured on a scale from 0 (representing no disability or full health) to 1 (representing death). Time lost, T, from a disease is measured in years. Life years lost are measured in relation to the greatest reported national life expectancy (that of Japanese women), something that is taken to be a measure of maximum possible life expectancy without disease. Hence the *burden* of a disease becomes the difference between a hypothetical maximum healthy life (disease free over a maximum possible remaining lifetime) and life lived untreated with disease. Acknowledging that the remaining lifetime if treated is shorter than Japanese life expectancy tables suggest, the *DALYs averted* as a consequence of intervention are less than the burden of the disease. Figure 13.6 (based on a figure in Fox-Rushby and Cairns, 2005) illustrates the difference between the disease burden and DALYs averted, and the similarities with the QALY concepts. The disease burden is the sum of the DALYs lost from disease and DALYs averted. Note also that DALYs averted are similar to QALYs gains, i.e. arithmetically the DALY is an inverted QALY.

The DALY has met with much criticism from QALY proponents. The heart of this criticism is related to the methodological short cuts used in the derivation of the disability weights. First, while the Q in the QALY is based on preferences held by patients or the public, the D in the DALY reflect person trade-off scores

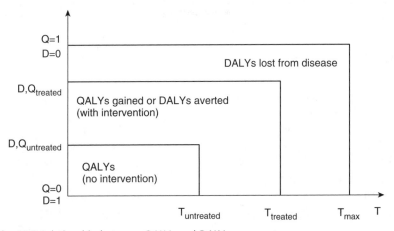

Fig. 13.6 Relationship between QALYs and DALYs.

from a small panel of health care workers. Second, the Q can take any value between 0 and 1 depending upon the particular health state, while the D has only seven disability weights. Hence, all health states are categorized into one out of seven alternative values. On this basis, it might therefore be appropriate to refer to the DALY as an *un*sophisticated *inverted* QALY!

13.2.3 **Comparing different measures of health outcome**

Most health outcome measures can be applied for the purpose of answering the basic medical question: to which extent is the new procedure better than the existing? However, very few outcome measures claim to be able to answer the basic health policy question: is it better to allocate health care resources on the treatment of patients with disease X or with disease Y?

Answering this question requires that the different degrees of health gains can be identified, measured, and then valued using a commensurable metric. Table 13.2 gives a summary of the various outcome measures discussed so far, in terms of their degree of commensurability as well as their basis for valuation (preference based or not). Uni-dimensional end points (e.g. infarction rates), as well as the multi-dimensional condition-specific descriptive systems, lose out on all four criteria, i.e. they are incommensurable and not preference based. Survival rate is an outcome measure that is commensurable regarding mortality only, while the so-called 'health profiles' are commensurable across morbidity only. QALYs emerge as the only measure of health effect that satisfies all four criteria, while DALYs lose out on the criterion 'preference based'.

Table 13.2 Types of health outcome measure depending on commensurability and basis for valuation (preference based or not)

	Commensurable across:			Preference based
	mortality, T	morbidity, Q	mortality and morbidity, Q*T	
Survival rates, increased life expectancy	Yes	No	No	No
Uni-dimensional end points; 'soft' or 'intermediate' Multi-dimensional condition-specific instruments	No	No	No	No
Health profiles, e.g. SF 36	No	Yes	No	No
QALYs (quality-adjusted life years)	Yes	Yes	Yes	Yes
DALYs (disability-adjusted life years)	Yes	Yes	Yes	No

There might be other classes of benefits from health care programmes beyond those identified as outcomes. These are the potential production gains as a consequence of improved health and 'process characteristics' beyond its consequences. In order to value these wider benefits, monetary-valuation techniques can be used.

Going back to the general Figure 13.1 on costs and effects, there are two distinctly different types of effect: health effects and production gains. As described above, health effects are normally measured in non-monetary terms. Since production gains are measured in monetary terms, these two types of effect cannot be aggregated: they are *incommensurable*. Before discussing how to value health in monetary terms in order to make it commensurable, let us consider the issues of how to measure, and how to account for, production gains within an economic evaluation.

13.3 Production gains resulting from improved health

There is still confusion in some parts of the economic evaluation literature about how to measure the economic benefits to society of a person's return to work as a consequence of their improved health. Some authors use gross income, some use net income, while others consider governmental savings in sickness benefits, and some suggest only to include the economic contributions to the rest of society. So, which types of economic benefits are there, and to whom?

In attempting to clarify these matters, it is crucial to distinguish between the *real changes* in the value of society's production and *transfer payments* across different agents in the economy. Table 13.3 illustrates what happens when a previously sick worker returns to work. Consider the three parties; the worker, the employer, and the government. The employer experiences a production gain, PG, attributable to the return of the worker, but the employer has to pay a wage, W, in return for the worker's productive efforts. The worker receives a net wage after taxation, T, but loses their sickness benefit, SB. The government receives taxation and gains from not having to pay sickness benefit. (In this case, the government acts as a social insurer, but the principle of transfer payments would hold under private insurance schemes as well.) Table 13.3 now illustrates how transfers are 'netted out' across the three parties. Thus, what remains is what matters: namely, the production gains.

The crucial message from Table 13.3 is the identification of production gains as the real economic changes, i.e. the effects on the national economy in terms of increased general domestic product (GDP). How do we measure these gains?

Table 13.3 The return of a productive worker: real production effects vs transfers

	Worker	Employer	Government
Increased production		+ PG	
Wage impacts	+ (W – T)	– W	+ T
Sickness benefits	– SB		+ SB

Under perfect competition in the labour market, the wage rate will reflect the value of the marginal product. Hence, in order to avoid the difficult task of measuring the productivity of each worker, the wage earned is often used as a proxy for production gains. Interestingly, the early literature on the value of human life used the wage rate as the basis for its estimation: the present value of remaining future gross earnings is referred to as *the human capital approach*.

The next issue is *how* this production gain is accounted for in a societal economic evaluation, i.e. within a cost—benefit analysis (CBA) and a cost-effectiveness analysis (CEA).

Figure 13.1 classified costs into health care costs (*HC*) and other resources. These other resource costs include different types of time costs, the largest item of which is the production *losses* (*PL*) whilst undergoing treatment. Within a *non*-welfare economic CBA (see Table 13.1), the benefit to society is measured as the increased production. The net present value (NPV), then, becomes the production gain (*PG*) minus all programme costs:

$$NPV = PG - (HC + PL) \tag{13.10}$$

Note that benefits from improved health per se are not included in this type of CBA. Within a CEA, the monetarized production gains cannot appear in the denominator together with *non*-monetarized units of health (remember: incommensurable units cannot be added!). *PG* will therefore appear in the numerator, like a cost saving to be subtracted in order to arrive at the 'net economic costs to society'. These net costs are then divided by the number of health benefit units (*H*) in order to derive a cost-effectiveness ratio for health:

$$CER_H = \frac{(HC + PL) - PG}{H} \tag{13.11}$$

The above formulae show the technical issue of how production gains are taken into account within CBA and CEA. Clearly, the higher the production gains, the better will the programme appear to society. In Equation 13.10, since only *net* economic benefits matter, the higher the production gains from treating a particular patient group, the more health care costs society would be prepared to tolerate. The same goes for the cost-effectiveness formula in Equation 13.11: since the cost-effectiveness ratio is concerned with the *net* societal costs, then the more production gains can be subtracted, the more favourable the ratio becomes.

This brings us from the *positive* issue of correctly assessing the magnitude of production gains to the *normative* issue of how much of these gains should be accounted for within a societal economic analysis. The dilemma in a priority-setting context is the implication that the most productive groups in society are being prioritized at the expense of groups who, for various reasons, are less productive. This implication, together with the methodological difficulties in how to correctly estimate the real production gains, explains why the inclusion of production gains has been a heated issue in the literature, and why many national guidelines for economic evaluations in health care object to their inclusion. Interestingly, the US panel that discussed guidelines for CEA argued for taking account of 'only the impact on the *rest* of society' (Weinstein *et al.*, 1997). In other words, taxes and voluntary contributions to the rest of society represent the types of gains believed to be relevant in a CEA.

This view that 'only the impact on the rest of society' matters resembles the concept of the 'breadwinner'. The breadwinner is important for the rest of the household to the extent that his revenues secure their feeding—with bread but also, hopefully, with other food. Therefore, a decisive issue when choosing whose life to save would be how important an individual is for the well-being of *other members* of the household or tribe. Hence, when constrained collective resources are being spent, it is the magnitude of the goods returned to the collective that matters, and not the net own income that the individual may legitimately keep to themselves.

For simplicity let us assume that all contributions to others are being channelled through taxation. Furthermore, assume a policy context in which all health care is tax financed. Hence, rather than including gross earning as the PG to be subtracted in the numerator of the CER, only that part of earnings that ends up as taxation is subtracted.

Consider the numerical examples in Table 13.4. This shows three alternative health care programmes (A, B, C), which yield identical health effect, H ($= 1$ QALY). The programmes differ in terms of health care costs (HC), production gains ($PG = W$), and taxation (T). Consequently, the cost-effectiveness ratios differ depending on whether, and which, gains are subtracted. If we take a 'narrow' perspective and account for health care costs only, programme A emerges as the most cost effective ($HC/H = 30$). If we take a broad perspective and account for the full production gains in the numerator, programme C becomes the most cost effective, $(HC - PG) / H = 5$. If we take a somewhat intermediate

Table 13.4 Cost-effectiveness ratios differ depending on whether, and which, gains are subtracted

H (QALY)		HC	PG	T	HC /H	(HC − PG)/H	(HC − T)/H
A	1	30	0	0	30	30	30
B	1	40	30	12	40	10	28
C	1	60	55	22	60	5	38

approach and account for tax contributions only, programme B is the most cost effective: $(HC - T)/H = 28$.

In principle, taxation serves three missions: i) social insurance for the taxpayer, ii) financing public goods and other government expenses, and iii) redistribution to other members of society. Therefore only a fraction will go to finance health care. Hence, if we prefer to take a 'health care resource implication' perspective when calculating the cost-effectiveness ratio, we would subtract only that fraction of T which is likely to end up as increased health care revenues.

There is no right or wrong answer to the question of whether, and how much, production gains should be taken into account within a health economic evaluation. There are two extreme views: ignore it all or include it all. An intermediate view in a policy context of tax-financed health care is to include only that fraction that ends up as tax contributions. Even so, policy makers may disapprove of the implication that—under proportional or progressive taxation—high-income-earning patient groups will be prioritized. An alternative position then would be to account for only that fraction of tax revenues that will end up as increased health care budgets. For example, with a tax rate of 40%, and with 20% of tax revenues for health care, 8% of the full production gains are taken into account.

If the analyses were concerned with changes in those resources that are under the control of 'the rest of society', which for simplicity can be seen as government, it follows that any changes in tax revenues or sickness payments become relevant (see Table 13.3). The public purse will save sickness benefits when previously ill people return to work, and these savings can be spent on more health care or more other publicly funded goods.[1] Again, although the implication is one of favouring patient groups that have a job to return to, other members of society may still approve of such a policy—as long as the

---

[1] For a theoretical discussion on the inclusion of taxes and sickness benefits, see Olsen and Richardson (1999).

treatment costs are less than the expected increased revenues and savings for the public purse.

13.4 The monetary value of improved health

In line with the view that people demand health care for its expected effects on health (Grossman, 1972), the focus here is on the monetary value of improved *health* rather than the monetary value of *health care*.

13.4.1 Valuing what

Improved health can vary in magnitude from the case of a saved infant with an expected remaining health span as in Figure 1.1, to a marginal fraction of a QALY that is too small to be illustrated in the figure. Hence, the more remaining *lifetime*, T, the higher the health gain; the larger the health state utility increment, Q, the higher the health gain; and the larger the probability, p, of a successful outcome from an intervention, the higher the expected health gain. Finally, the more patients, N, that can be treated, the higher the health gain. That more is better in terms of health gains not only makes intuitive sense, but it is stated in policy objectives as well, such as 'maximizing health gains'. We would therefore require that when valuing health gains in *monetary* terms, the valuation instrument should pick up variations in the size of the health effects. In other words, the larger the T, Q, p or N, the higher the monetary value of the health care programme. If not, I would conclude that the instrument fails its most important validity test.

13.4.2 Valuing how

In general, preferences can be *revealed* from actual behaviour in markets, where trade-offs are made across different goods with different attributes. Alternatively, consumers can *state* their preferences through choices presented to them in hypothetical questions.

In general, economists favour revealed preferences, because they put more faith in how people *actually* behave than in how people *say* they would behave. This principle is fine in situations where markets provide the goods, but when the goods that we want to value are not available in ordinary markets, preferences would have to be elicited in other ways. Rarely would we find market analogues through which consumers have had the opportunity to signal their values of health improvements.

As far as the feasibility of inferring consumers' monetary values from revealed behaviour is concerned, the value of safety appears to occupy a middle ground between 'normal goods' and health. A range of safety features is available in the market (e.g. safer cars, smoke detectors), and by dividing the price of a safety feature by its marginal risk reduction, an *implicit value of life* can be inferred. Comparisons of such estimates of implicit values of life show huge variations across different types of risk-reducing goods (see Tengs *et al.*, 1995). Thus, consumers are either misinformed about the magnitude of various risk reductions and/or they have very clear views on how they would prefer *not* to die. Another market analogue from which a monetary value of life can be revealed is the labour market, in which increasing wages are used as compensation for accepting increasing risks.

For goods that are not available in well-functioning markets, or for which market analogues are hard to find, economists have developed methods for constructing *hypothetical markets*. These methods are termed *contingent valuation*, whereby respondents are asked to express a value that would be true under certain specified conditions. Contingent valuation is an umbrella term for different types of hypothetical monetary valuation questions. By far the most widely applied version of contingent valuation in health and health care is the willingness-to-pay (WTP) method.

The logical starting point in a WTP study is to specify what exactly is being valued. A key concept here is the *scenario description* that explains the characteristics of the particular good. For health care, it is important to describe types of outcomes, i.e. any improvements in health state, its duration, and the probability of success. If framed in an ex ante insurance context, the probability of needing the service represents a crucial piece of information. If framed in a public policy context, the number of patients being treated by the health care programme is an important piece of information. In addition, any other description about the process of treatment should be included if it is believed to be relevant. Ideally, information on all the assumed utility-yielding attributes of the programme should be provided—including any disutility-yielding side effects. However, the cognitive capacity of respondents obviously represents a constraint on exactly how much information can be dealt with.

A second issue, and one that has attracted much interest, is the question format, i.e. how the WTP question should be phrased. There are four alternatives: i) *open ended*, which basically asks 'How much would you be willing to pay?' without giving any reference sum; ii) *closed ended*, which asks 'Would you be willing to pay X dollars?', where X is varied across sub-samples and a demand curve is estimated based on how the proportion of yes-respondents varies across sub-samples; iii) *iterative bidding games*, whereby the interviewer starts with a specified bid and follows up by asking if higher or lower sums would be acceptable depending on the answer to the preceding bid; and iv) *payment cards*, where alternative sums are listed, usually from 0 to a realistic maximum, and where respondents are asked to circle the amount which comes closest to their maximum WTP. In this literature, different camps hold fairly strong views on which question format is the best or most correct. However, the degree of scientific attention to this methodological issue does not seem to correspond with its applied importance in terms of the relative differences in mean values that the methods seem to produce.

13.4.3 **Theoretical attraction and practical problems**

Among mainstream economists, the primary attraction of the willingness-to-pay method is its roots in neoclassical welfare economics, i.e. it is 'theoretically correct'! This assertion that the method is 'theoretically correct' seems more like tautology than an argument or reason. Still, the welfare economic paradigm includes some appealing assumptions about consumer preferences: consumers are the best judge of their own welfare; they have preferences over all imaginable goods no matter how hypothetical; and they make trade-offs between own income and increasing quantities of the good.

The WTP is founded on the dictum that a good has *value* to a consumer only to the extent that they are prepared to *sacrifice* something in order to obtain it. So, the more they are willing to sacrifice of their own income, the higher the value of the good in question. The maximum WTP would then express the respondent's valuation of the good in monetary terms. A crucial assumption here is that of 'more is better' (up to a meaningful satiation level), i.e. the larger the quantity of the particular good, the more income the consumer is prepared to sacrifice. While many of us have experienced satiation points for ordinary consumption goods ('I don't want more chocolate now'), it is hard to envisage the existence of satiation for health gains, whether for ourselves or other people: more *health* is *always* better!

WTP is fine in theory but unfortunately problematic in practice. Beattie *et al.* (1998) suggested that WTP answers are 'sensitive to theoretically *ir*relevant factors, and *in*sensitive to theoretically relevant factors'. Probably the most important *relevant* factor is the size of the good: people should be willing to pay more for more. But there is much evidence that WTP is insensitive to the magnitude of such things as the size of the risk reduction and the scope of the benefit. And there is now some supporting evidence from the health field, which shows that WTP is insensitive to the size of health outcomes (see e.g. Olsen *et al.*, 2004). Hence, this valuation instrument fails a most important validity test.

Examples of theoretically *ir*relevant factors include the fact that slight changes in the wording of scenario descriptions can have dramatic effects on stated WTP and the finding that the respondent's valuation of a preceding programme can affect their value of a subsequent programme. When the most significant determinant of a respondent's WTP for programme B is their WTP for a previously valued (and completely different) programme A, their valuation cannot be *independent of irrelevant alternatives*, and doubt must again be cast on the reliability of WTP responses.

13.5 **Threshold values and net monetary benefits**

A fairly recent use of the term WTP in the economic evaluation literature is to denote an explicit threshold value of a QALY, or an implied value that represents an upper level for accepted cost effectiveness as *society's willingness to pay for a QALY*. In some countries, a health governing body (e.g. NICE in the UK) has stated explicit (ranges of) threshold values. If the incremental cost-effectiveness ratio (ICER) is above the threshold value, the new programme will not be accepted. If the ICER is below the threshold, the programme will receive public funding. Hence, the threshold value tells how much society is prepared to pay for a QALY, i.e. *society's willingness to pay*. If threshold values are not stated in health policy documents, one might alternatively inquire into past decisions within a government body that makes similar recommendations, such as pharmaceutical benefit advisory committees. The highest ICER that has been accepted would then be inferred as an implied maximum WTP for a QALY.

This use of the WTP term is different from a welfare economic connotation, which requires that WTP values reflect individual preferences as stated in contingent valuation studies. Therefore researchers are now attempting to elicit WTP per QALY gained directly from individuals. An important research question is the extent to which individual preferences correspond with society's threshold values.

Provided that a cost-effectiveness threshold value, (T_V), or a WTP per QALY has been established, then a programme with an ICER below this threshold will provide a net benefit to society. Based on the simple logic that the T_V tells the benefit of a QALY, while the ICER tells how much it costs, a rearrangement of terms will bring us from a cost-effectiveness expression to a cost—benefit expression:

$$\Delta C/\Delta E < T_V \Rightarrow T_V \Delta E - \Delta C > 0 \tag{13.12}$$

This is referred to as the *net monetary benefit*, NMB, from the programme:

$$NMB = T_V \Delta E - \Delta C \tag{13.13}$$

Hence, T_V represents the monetary *value* of each unit of effectiveness, ΔE represents the incremental health effects (QALYs) from the programme, while

ΔC represents the incremental costs of the programme. It follows that if the ICER exceeds the threshold value, the net monetary benefit is negative.

The idea of one threshold value is put forward as an argument for consistent decision making, something which makes sense if the health policy objective was uni-dimensional health maximization. However, since most health policy objectives include concerns for equity and fairness as well as the size of total health gains (the twin objective of efficiency and equity), it follows that the value of a QALY will have to differ depending on how it scores in terms of equity. Hence, the urge for *one* threshold value is a delusion!

13.6 **Conclusion**

The rationale for spending money on health care is to improve people's health. The challenge is how to *identify*, *measure*, and *value* different types of health improvements. For the purpose of making comparisons across programme areas, health outcomes must be valued in a *commensurable* metric. Returning to Table 13.1, three of the four boxes involve a commensurable metric: the two boxes using a monetary valuation and the non-monetary preference-based combination. The methodologies used in these three boxes are productivity measures, willingness to pay, and QALYs. Production gains, however, do not represent a metric for valuing improved health per se, but rather the economic *consequences* of improved health.

When valuing the improved health in monetary terms, there is a danger of double counting the production gains, i.e. that the respondent may have included the utility of increased income associated with good health when stating their willingness-to-pay value. However, it is unlikely that the respondent has accounted for the benefits from that part of their production gains that accrue to other members of society, i.e. their tax contributions.

There is much empirical evidence to suggest that individuals value health care for more than its outcomes or that the process of care matters. However, the *relative* value of process characteristics compared with the value of health outcomes is harder to measure. Furthermore, consumers of health care are likely to express different trade-offs between process vs outcome attributes than the same individuals would express in the role of taxpayers (see also Chapter 3, section 3.2.2).

Valuing health benefits in monetary terms has the theoretical advantage of making benefits commensurable, not only across other types of benefits, but with costs as well. However, there are severe methodological problems involved in eliciting valid and reliable WTP values. QALYs represent a more limited metric, in that they are not commensurable with costs. Hence, they are used in cost-effectiveness analyses rather than cost—benefit analyses. In both types of analysis, though, measuring costs is required, to which we will now turn.

Suggested reading

Brazier, J., Ratcliffe, J., Salamon, J. A. and Tsuchiya, A. (2007) *Measuring and valuing health benefits for economic evaluation*. Oxford: Oxford University Press.

Lloyd, A. J. (2003) Threats to the estimation of benefit: are preference elicitation methods accurate? *Health Economics*, 12, 393–402.

Gyrd-Hansen, D. (2005) Willingness to pay for a QALY: theoretical and methodological issues. *PharmacoEconomics*, 23 (5), 423–32.

Exercises

1. Find out which types of health outcome measures are recommended in various national guidelines for economic evaluations. See http://www.ispor.org/peguidelines/index.asp

2. Choose a diagnosis—treatment pair (e.g. depression—antidepressant medication) that interests you, and find out which type of health outcome measures (see Table 13.2) have been most commonly used in studies in which the treatment effectiveness has been documented.

3. See the EQ-5D descriptive system, and imagine yourself in the health state described as combination [21221] http://www.euroqol.org/. Ask yourself the VAS, TTO, SG and PTO questions. To which extents do the implied health-state values from your answers differ, and why do you think they differ in the ways they do?

Chapter 14

Costs and discounting

This chapter explores the other two key parameters in the cost—benefit and cost-effectiveness formulae; how to measure costs, and the principle of discounting. While cost calculations may sound like a boring technical exercise, discounting health effects is more of a controversial normative issue.

If you think that number of patients treated is important when deciding which health care programmes to prioritize, then by implication you will think that taking cost into consideration is important! With a given sum of money to allocate, the higher the treatment costs, the fewer patients can be treated. This is why we need to learn some basics when it comes to estimating costs. And if you wonder why future costs and effects are valued less when they occur in the future, and how this is calculated, then you need to learn about discounting.

14.1 Average vs marginal costs

Probably the most cited example of the practical importance of marginal cost information for health care resource allocation is the study of the costs of guaiac stool testing (Neuhauser and Lewicki, 1975). Based on the suggested guidelines by medical specialists, six sequential tests were recommended for detecting cancer in the bowel. If all six tests were performed, the average cost was estimated at $2,451 per detected cancer. However, because the incremental detection rate diminished strongly with each additional test, the marginal cost was $47 million per detected case from performing the sixth test. While this extreme difference between marginal and average costs has been questioned, the important message from this example is that average cost figures are a misleading basis for determining cost consequences of marginal changes in an activity. This highlights the importance of information about marginal costs when making resource allocation decisions.

As with the distinction between fixed and variable input factors (see Chapter 2), there is a distinction between fixed and variable costs. *Fixed costs* are the costs of fixed input factors, such as investment in buildings and machinery. These costs do not vary with the quantity produced. *Variable costs*, on the other hand, vary with the level of output. They include the costs of such input factors as labour, energy, and raw materials. The more we decide to produce, the more of such input factors are required. Total costs, *TC*, are then fixed costs, *FC*, plus variable costs, *VC*, the latter being a function of quantity, *X*:

$$TC = FC + V(X) \tag{14.1}$$

Average costs, *AC*, are simply the result of dividing total costs by the given quantity:

$$AC = TC / X \tag{14.2}$$

Note that when dividing fixed costs by the quantity produced, these average fixed costs will fall with increasing levels of production. If variable costs are completely linear with the increasing level of production, the average variable costs are constant. Hence, the more we produce, the cheaper it becomes per unit—a situation referred to as 'economies of scale'. However, the relationship between variable input factors and level of production is more complicated than such a simple one-to-one-relationship.

The explanation for a non-linear relationship between variable costs and output can be found by returning to Figure 2.1, which illustrates the typical relationship between one input factor and output. Note that beyond some level of production, average productivity will start to *decrease*. Logically, when the cost per unit of input factor is the same no matter how many people we employ, the average cost will start to *increase*.

Marginal costs, *MC*, are the additional costs following a one-unit change in production. Since fixed costs by definition remain unchanged, it is only the additional *variable* costs that matter:

$$MC = V(X + 1) - V(X) \tag{14.3}$$

When production increases by a step as a consequence of one extra worker employed, marginal costs are computed within the specific interval; the increased variable costs are divided by the increased units produced.

Figure 14.1 shows the general relationship between the average and marginal cost curves. Fixed average costs (*FC / X*) are always decreasing with

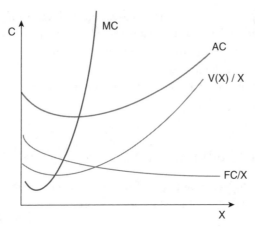

Fig. 14.1 Average and marginal costs.

increasing X. Variable average costs $(V(X) / X)$ follow a U-shaped pattern. Total average costs (AC) are at their lowest when the decrease in fixed variable costs outweigh the increase in variable average costs—a production level referred to as *technical optimum*.

As long as marginal costs are lower than average costs, average costs will fall. Average costs will increase when marginal costs are higher than average costs. Hence, the MC curve will always intersect the AC curve at its lowest point, i.e. in the *technical optimum*.

Which production level is the best? If we are concerned only about costs, the technical optimum is the best because this is where average costs are at their lowest. However, if the aim is to maximize profit, i.e. revenues minus costs, the producer must compare the marginal revenue from the last unit sold (i.e. the price) with the cost of producing it (i.e. the marginal cost). Hence, the best production level for a profit-maximizing firm is where price equals marginal costs, provided of course that this is beyond the technical optimum.

Hospitals that are *not* motivated by profit maximization might also find it relevant to compare their marginal costs of treating an additional patient with the revenues received for doing so. Under activity-based financing, hospitals are reimbursed at prices equal to the national average costs of the various diagnosis—treatment pairs. If marginal costs exceed this average cost price, then in isolation the last unit will involve a loss that has to be compensated from other sources of revenues. If hospitals consistently provide services at higher marginal costs than the price, they end up with deficits.

There is a saying that 'the only relevant costs are those from which you can escape'. If a producer is forced to reduce its production, it cannot escape the fixed costs—only some variable costs. Interestingly, some types of costs are more variable when considering *increased* activity than when considering *reduced* activity. Labour laws in many countries make it more difficult to sack workers than to employ new workers. Hence, labour costs are variable with respect to expansions, but to some extent fixed with respect to contractions.

Costs in a hospital ward

This example is based on the relationship between labour input, L, and output, X, from Table 2.1 in Chapter 2. Assume that labour unit cost is 200 and fixed costs are 1,000.

Fixed average costs (FC / X) decrease with increasing X; variable average costs (VC / X) decrease until $X = 28$, and start increasing after $X = 35$; and total average costs (TC / X) are at their lowest when $X = 40$.

Compare Table 2.1 and note that average variable costs fall as long as average productivity increases. When average productivity starts to decrease, average variable costs will start to increase. The last column of the table represents the marginal costs. The third worker is the most productive (increasing X from 10 to 20), and would therefore contribute to the lowest marginal costs $(200 / 10 = 20)$. The seventh worker employed has the lowest marginal productivity, implying the highest marginal costs $(200 / 2 = 100)$.

Table 14.1 Average costs and marginal costs

X	FC	VC= (200*L)	TC	$\frac{FC}{X}$	$\frac{VC}{X}$	$\frac{TC}{X}$	$\frac{\Delta VC}{\Delta X}$ =MC
0	1000	0	1000	∞	0	∞	
4	1000	200	1200	250	50	300	50
10	1000	400	1400	100	40	140	33
20	1000	600	1600	50	30	80	20
28	1000	800	1800	36	29	64	25
35	1000	1000	2000	29	29	57	29
40	1000	1200	2200	25	30	55	40
42	1000	1400	2400	24	33	57	100

Exercise: put the numbers from the last four columns into a figure like Figure 14.1.

14.2 **Identifying cost items: analysis viewpoint**

Some early health economics literature made a distinction between direct and indirect costs, the former referring to health care, the latter to costs in other sectors, most notably the production consequences for the rest of the economy. This distinction was misleading: which costs are interpreted as 'direct' and which as 'indirect' crucially depend on the viewpoint of the analysis. More 'viewpoint-neutral' terms can be found in recent literature when referring to cost types such as health care costs, travel costs, etc. However, there is still some confusion when it comes to production consequences. Do they refer to production *losses* related to time away from work whilst being treated or to production *gains* following improved health? Note that the former is a cost, while the latter is an effect or a monetary benefit, as we discussed in Chapter 13.

Which cost items should be included? A narrow analysis would take the perspective of the producer and consider only those costs that the producer is faced with—defined as *private* costs. Logically, such analysis neglects any cost consequences on other institutions. As a minimum a health economic cost appraisal would include the costs of all health service institutions, e.g. not only treatment costs in hospital but also costs related to follow-up consultations in primary care.

Beyond the health sector, there are other related sectors that may face costs. In the UK, for example, with its publicly financed national health service, the *Guide to the method of technology appraisal* suggests including the 'resource costs and savings for the NHS and personal social services (PSS)'. Costs to other government bodies may be reported separately in 'exceptional circumstances', i.e. if 'a substantial proportion of the costs (or cost savings) are expected to be incurred outside the NHS and PSS' (www.nice.org.uk). Such a costing methodology takes the perspective of the public sector rather than of wider society.

In addition to the cost consequences that appear on public sector accounts, there may be costs to patients and their families, and to other private sector accounts as well. A comprehensive economic evaluation will consider the full resource implications for society as a whole, i.e. it will identify *all* cost items regardless of which accounts they appear on.

The first step is to identify which cost items to include, the next is to measure how many units of each cost item, C_j, are required, and the next is to value them: $V_j^* C_j$. A problem with the last step is that either market prices might not be available or they might not reflect the actual limited availability of the resources.

14.3 **Health service costs**

Over 70% of hospital costs are labour costs. So if we are considering the cost of a particular medical procedure, we can start by counting how many personnel are required for how many hours. If we multiply each personnel group's total hours by its wage rates, we can expect to measure about three-quarters of its costs. In addition to the direct treatment costs, there are 'indirect overhead costs' that stem from hospital administration and support facilities. Different criteria can be used for distributing these shared costs.

An alternative to undertaking a detailed estimation of all cost items would be to apply national average costs from a DRG tariff. If labour productivities and wages are similar across the country, such average cost figures may be a sound basis for *long-run* decisions about investments and capacity planning in the hospital. Marginal costs, however, are still the most relevant basis for making *short-term* activity decisions.

In addition to hospital costs, there may be follow-up costs in primary care and rehabilitation institutions. Clearly, these are relevant cost items that must be measured and valued. A more contentious issue is the extent to which future health care costs should be accounted for. If the future health care costs are *related* to the particular intervention, it seems highly appropriate to include them as would any other follow-up activity. However, if the future health care costs are *unrelated* to the particular intervention or condition, they should *not* be included as an additional cost item. Although a saved life will involve additional expected costs to the health sector during the gained life years lived, the use of these future resources will follow as a consequence of a *future* health state. Spending resources to improve that particular *future* health state should be justified by the expected health effects of those resources, something which should be based on a *separate* economic evaluation of the costs and effects of the specific future intervention.

14.4 **Non-health service costs**

Patients often face costs related to their treatment. If they live far from the hospital or the GP, *travel costs* are involved. In addition, there are *time costs*, based on the premise that time always has alternative uses. If leisure time is sacrificed, the conventional way is to value it by net income. Based on the model for income—leisure trade-off (Figure 10.3) it follows that the marginal leisure time has an alternative value in the *net income* forgone.

If working time is sacrificed, *gross income* earned during the time away is the standard method for valuing the production loss to society. *Production losses* represent a potentially big cost component, particularly for screening programmes that include large groups of people from the labour force who lose productive time at work. Hence the more the individual earns, the more it costs to screen them!

An issue that has raised debate in the literature is how to deal with indirect taxation, i.e. should value added tax (VAT) be included when estimating costs? The argument for *excluding* VAT is that taxation is a transfer payment that does not reflect real costs of scarce resources. An argument for *including* VAT follows a welfare-economic logic related to how the benefit side should be valued in a cost—benefit analysis (CBA): when benefits are expressed through willingness to pay (WTP), such benefits reflect people's willingness to sacrifice other goods, and these other goods are being valued at a rate that includes VAT. Hence, if the estimation of costs in a CBA is based on the same methodology as in a CEA, cost figures should include VAT. Whichever argument you find more compelling, always make clear whether VAT has been included or not (and of course the rate of VAT).

14.5 **The discount rate**

Discounting reflects a preference for the present. A discount rate is used as a 'time weighting' to devalue the future: the stronger the preference for the present, the higher the time weighting. In health economic evaluations, the idea of discounting is controversial because it implies that future health gains are assigned lower social values than current health gains. An important question is whether health benefits should be discounted at a different rate from costs, i.e. should we use a lower rate for health in the denominator than in the numerator of the cost-effectiveness ratio? Answering 'no' to this accepts the 'eternal delay' implications of health investments. If the rate of decline of costs is greater than that for benefits, no programme would be undertaken within the current period because the cost per unit of benefit would always be less next period. However, this 'paralysing paradox' relates to budget allocation over time. If health planners have no scope for deferring current funds to future periods, then the idea of deferring all health care resources to the infinite future is irrelevant. Interestingly, previous UK guidelines suggested a discount rate of 6% on costs and 2.5% on health effects.

There are two different reasons for applying a positive discount rate for public projects. First, there is the argument referred to as 'the social opportunity cost of capital': the rate of return on public projects should ideally be the same as the marginal private project that is being forgone. Second, because consumers have a preference for the present, they claim compensation for delaying consumption; the rate of this compensation is their *time-preference rate*.

Individuals' time preferences represent the aggregate of three distinct inter-temporal concerns: pure time preference, which refers solely to remoteness in time and thus reflects degree of impatience; the rate at which the marginal util-ity of increased future consumption diminishes; and uncertainty.

14.5.1 Formulae and examples

The mathematical formulae are fairly simple as long as we operate with a con-stant discount rate, r, and discrete time. The present value of an item, Z, with a unitary value of 1, occurring at a given future time, t, is:

$$Z_{PVt} = \frac{1}{(1+r)^t} \tag{14.5}$$

It follows that the larger the discount rate and the further into the future we look, the higher becomes the denominator and, thus, the lower is the present value, Z_{PVt}. With this formula, we get the present value of a given number of health benefits that occur in a future time period, t.

If the benefits occur as a constant stream every year during the programme period, the present value of this stream is considered as an annuity. The for-mula for this annuity, A, with a unitary value of 1 (due at the end of each year) throughout the period, t, is:

$$A = \frac{1}{(1+r)} + \frac{1}{(1+r)^2} + \frac{1}{(1+r)^3} + \cdots + \frac{1}{(1+r)^t} = \frac{1-(1+r)^{-t}}{r} \tag{14.6}$$

Table 14.2 shows the effects of different discount rates. A zero discount rate implies the same value to an event no matter how far into the future it occurs. A 10% rate could be used because it reflects time preferences for health (in fact, some empirical studies have found rates in excess of 10%). A rate of 5% used

Table 14.2 Some examples of the present values of a future event, Z_{PVt}, and a stream of events, A, depending on the discount rate, r, and time, t

	Z_{PVt}		A	
r	$t = 5$	$t = 20$	$t = 5$	$t = 20$
0%	1	1	5	20
3%	0.86	0.55	4.6	14.9
5%	0.78	0.38	4.3	12.5
10%	0.62	0.15	3.8	8.5

to be the standard rate in applied economic evaluations of health care. More recently, the standard rate has been reduced to 3%, which is now the recommended rate for economic evaluations in many countries, including the USA, Sweden and Italy.

The higher the discount rate, r, the less weight is given to health gains occurring in the future compared with health gains occurring now. In addition, the further into a future time period, t, the larger the impact of discounting. If a 10% rate is used, a life saved in five years is *devalued* to 0.62 of one life saved today, while a life saved in 20 years' time is *devalued* to only 0.15 compared with one life saved today. Therefore, the health policy relevance of the discounting issue becomes more important for long-term preventive programmes than for curative ones. When discounting over the course of an individual's *lifetime*, the annuity columns show how life years are devalued, e.g. using a 3% discount rate implies that 20 life years count for only 14.9 years in present-value terms. Figure 14.2 illustrates how the discount rate affects the magnitudes of the present value of 20 discounted life years gained. The rectangular box represents 20 *un*discounted life years. The darkest area shows the present value stream if we apply a 10% annual discount rate. The areas under the 5% curve and the 3% curve illustrate the respective remaining present values.

Clearly, the further into the future we consider, the more the benefits will disappear as a consequence of discounting. If you discount a full life of 75 years using 3%, it reduces to a present value of 30 discounted life years!

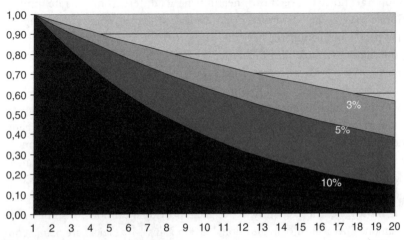

Fig. 14.2 The present value of 20 life years gained, based on discount rates of 3%, 5%, and 10%.

14.5.2 **Some views on discounting**

There are essentially three different normative views about how health should be discounted. First, we can use the same rate as for other goods in the economy. This argument emphasizes that capital allocated to health care has the same social opportunity cost as capital for other sectors. Accordingly, for consistency reasons, health gains should be subject to the same inter-temporal criteria as other goods. Second, we can use a zero rate or close to zero. Some medical ethicists hold that a life's value is the same no matter when it is saved, and a QALY would similarly be equally valued whether it is gained this year or in the distant future. According to this moral principle, that all generations should be given equal weight, it follows that health gains should be left undiscounted in economic evaluations.

Third, there is the view that we should use the rate that best corresponds with people's preferences. This is the view held by economists with an affinity to the consumer sovereignty principle. However, many economists have been uneasy about individuals' impatience for own consumption. The famous British welfare economist Arthur Pigou (1877–1959) held that the pure time preference reflects a human defect: 'our telescopic faculty is defective'. Since future pleasure will be no lower than present pleasure, society should therefore not take human impatience into account when determining a discount rate.

Given that individuals as citizens may have different time preferences for goods in a social context from those revealed in the context of private consumption, it might well be the case that the rate implied from an inter-temporal choice between own health benefits differs from the rate implied from a societal inter-temporal health choice. Moreover, some studies suggest that people (and animals!) have *decreasing timing aversion*, i.e. they attach less importance to a fixed time difference the further into the future the difference moves. As a consequence, so-called hyperbolic discounting models for health have been developed (see e.g. Cairns and van der Pol, 1997).

Within a health context, the discount rate is sometimes perceived as an inter-temporal *equity weight* that assigns relative social values to health gains depending on when they occur. Assuming constant technology over time, a discount rate of zero might be the most equitable, in that each generation counts the same. However, as opposed to such *inter*-generational considerations, the impact of the discount rate leads to the opposite conclusion regarding *intra*-generational equity. Since each individual cannot 'consume' more than one QALY each year, additional health gains—by logic—are being 'consumed' over time. A methodological solution to a preference for more equal distribution of health gains across patient groups is to apply a positive discount rate that assigns lower values to increasing number of QALYs. Hence, the stronger the preference for equal distribution of gains, the higher the discount rate.

14.6 **Conclusion**

In general, resources are scarce and will therefore always have alternative uses (see Chapter 2). The same goes for health care; that is why it is crucial to value how much of these resources are required for a new treatment programme. But what is so special about health care costs compared with other resource costs? First, there is a clear-cut opportunity cost in terms of forgone health improvements: when health care (e.g. doctors' time) is devoted to one particular patient group, it will not be available for another patient group. For non-health care resources, the alternative use would most likely *not* be health-enhancing activities, e.g. production losses imply fewer goods of value to society, but not necessarily less population health. Second, many societies have explicit equity objectives related to their distribution of health care resources but not for the other types of goods whose availability is affected by production losses.

Interestingly, estimation of costs is often considered to be a more value-free venture than estimation of health outcomes. But with costs, as with outcomes, analysts still have scope for manipulation. If the vested interest is to make a new procedure look cheap, clearly the analyst could try to neglect those cost components that are not immediately visible. While trained economists surely hold different views on the relevance of including various cost components, they nevertheless agree that it is correct—as well as honest—to present a transparent costing assessment, i.e. assessing which items in which quantities at which unit values.

Discounting health effects is something most economists would consider obvious in order to adjust for the different timings of when they occur. Nevertheless, the implication of 'devaluing' future health gains is something with which most non-economists are unfamiliar, e.g. when applying the current standard rate of 3%, a programme that is expected to save 100 lives in 20 years will give 56 'discounted lives' in the CE denominator; and if a programme increases life expectancy by 20 years for one person, it counts for only 14.9 'discounted years' in the denominator (see Table 14.2). Hence, a seemingly technical issue (the r in the formulae) has controversial normative implications in terms of how society values future health gains compared with current gains. It is time to discuss further such implicit and explicit distributive issues.

The early health economics literature on cost—benefit and cost-effectiveness analyses stressed that such analyses should be considered *an aid to decision making*, meaning that it is for decision makers to consider if—and which—additional issues beyond costs and effects should be taken into account.

Suggested reading

Drummond, M. F., Sculpher, M. J., Torrance, G. W., O'Brien, B. J. and Stoddart, G. L. (2005) *Methods for the Economic Evaluation of Health Care Programmes*. Oxford: Oxford University Press.

Leister, J. and Stausberg, J. (2004) Comparison of cost accounting methods from different DRG systems and their effect on health care quality. *Health Policy*, 74 (1), 46–55.

Cairns, J. (2001) Discounting in economic evaluation. In *Economic evaluation in health care: Merging theory with practice* (ed. M. Drummond and A. McGuire). Oxford: Oxford University Press.

Exercises

1. Go back to Table 14.1 and change FC (fixed costs) from 1000 to 200. Change the column figures accordingly. Which implications will the lower FC have on i) the technical optimum, and ii) marginal costs? Explain.

2. Explain the costing principles on which DRGs (diagnosis-related groups) are based.

3. Why should future health gains be discounted in an economic evaluation—or why should they not?

Chapter 15

Equity issues: going beyond CBA and ICER

This final chapter discusses distributive implications of some parameters *inside* the economic evaluation formulae, as well as some priority-relevant issues that lie *outside* these formulae. It is argued that an economic evaluation should always be complemented by a description of the equity implications of the programme. For this purpose an 'equity checklist' is suggested.

A characteristic feature of economic evaluation methodologies is their prospective nature. *Retrospective* issues are ignored, such as asking how much health patients have already had (their age, duration of suffering), as well as raising the controversial issue of the *cause* of their illness. Such issues, however, are often brought into the priority-setting debate. Before going outside the formulae, consider first the problem of income-dependent measures of benefits.

15.1 Productivity changes and willingness to pay vary with income

The blunt fact that productivity changes and willingness to pay vary with income is only a 'problem' in health policy settings that are guided by an objective of 'equal access for equal need, independent of income'. However, since this objective is a standard one in most publicly funded health care systems, the problem is a real one.

The standard way of measuring *production gains* is the 'human capital approach', which assigns a monetary value to human life according to the individual's productive capacity, measured by the present value of remaining future gross earnings. Clearly, the more someone earns, and the more time they have left in the workforce, the higher their human capital. In a much-cited study based on US data in 1967, the highest human capital was estimated for white men aged 30–34, with at least 16 years' education ($223,500), while the lowest was for coloured men above 85 years of age ($400).[1] By implication, when taking such benefits into account—either as a stand-alone benefit measure in a cost—benefit analysis or as an economic gain to be subtracted in the numerator of a cost-effectiveness analysis—this is at odds with the above-mentioned objective that access be independent of income. Because of the inequitable distributive implications of accounting for production gains, economic evaluation guidelines in many countries require that such 'indirect costs' are reported separately.

Willingness to pay (WTP) is used for estimating monetary values of improved health per se, not just the economic consequences of improved health. The absolute amount one is willing to sacrifice is taken to reflect one's strength of preferences—'a dollar is a dollar is a dollar'. Since rich people generally experience lower utility loss of their marginal sacrificed dollar than do poor people of their marginal sacrificed dollar, a given WTP will signal higher marginal utility for the poor than the same WTP would signal for the rich.

When respondents' WTP depends on how much they are *able* to sacrifice, it is a standard validity test in WTP studies to explore if WTP correlates with respondents' income. And it does—usually. Hence, health care programmes preferred by high income earners will be seen to yield high social benefits.

This income bias would not be a problem if there were no systematic income-related differences in disease patterns, and thus in *needs* for different types of health care. In practice, however, there are quite strong socio-economic variations in health. Therefore, if health care resource allocation were to be based on WTP values, there would be a bias towards those programmes favoured by high income earners. In other words, the value of a health care programme depends on how much money the individual is able to sacrifice in order to obtain it, rather than how much health improvement it can produce (see also the discussion in Chapter 9 related to Figure 9.3).

Economists who are trained within the paradigm of neoclassical welfare economics may instinctively think that the objective of the health service is to maximize social welfare, in terms of aggregated individual WTP.

[1] Rice, D. and Cooper, B. (1967) The economic value of human life. *American Journal of Public Health*, 57, 1954–66.

However, this *welfarist maximand* is quite different from the stated twin objectives of most publicly funded health services, namely: i) maximize population *health* (rather than welfare), and ii) equal access to health care for the purpose of reduced inequality in health. This alternative paradigm is often referred to as *non-welfarist* or extra-welfarist. In Chapter 4, the twin objectives were incorporated within a health-related social welfare function, and illustrated by a trade-off between efficiency as health maximization and equality in health gains.

15.2 **Health gains: size and distribution matter**

Preferences for equal distribution of health gains imply diminishing social value of increasing units of health gains. In cost-effectiveness analyses the health gains in the denominator of the incremental cost-effectiveness ratio (ICER) are valued linearly. What matters is the cost per *unit* of health outcomes, independent of the size of this outcome: e.g. € 500,000 for 10 QALYs and € 5,000 for 0.1 QALY are both recalculated to an ICER of € 50,000 per QALY. However, while everybody would agree about linearity in the numerator, i.e. that € 500,000 represents 100 times as much as € 5,000, the question is whether we agree with the assumption of linearity in the denominator, i.e. do we *value* 10 QALYs gained 100 times as much as 0.1 QALY gained? If people do not value QALYs gained linearly, cost-effectiveness analyses are not consistent with people's preferences.

There is empirical evidence to suggest that, over large health gains, people assign diminishing marginal value to increasing units of gains, e.g. 5 QALYs to each of four patients is better than 20 QALYs to one patient. Interestingly, such preferences can be accounted for when health gains are being discounted. Table 14.2 shows that, when using a discount rate of 5%, the present value of 20 years gained to one patient reduces to 12.5 discounted life years, which is less than the present values of 5 years' gain to each of three patients ($4.3*3 =$ 12.9). Or, put differently, the present value of the additional 15 (20 − 5) life years to one person has about the same value as the present value of the first 5 years to each of two persons.

At the other end of the scale—small health gains—recent studies suggest increasing marginal value of increasing units of small health gains, e.g. 5 years to one patient is better than 1 month to each of 60 patients. Hence, rather than a simplistic linear valuation of health gains, our preferences might better be expressed through an S-shaped function that allows for the existence of a *lower threshold* below which we care less, as well as an *upper threshold* above which we care less.

What matters in the current context of equity issues in economic evaluation is the existence of an *upper* threshold—or a diminishing marginal value of increasing QALYs to the same beneficiary. The rate at which increasing health gains should be diminished can be expressed in terms of a discount rate, or an equity parameter in the health-related social welfare function (see Chapter 4).

15.3 Severity: equality in prospective health

With its pure focus on *incremental* gains, ΔE, the ICER disregards any differences in what is being subtracted, e.g. adding 2 months of life to a patient who will otherwise die, or to someone who will otherwise expect to live another 10 years does not matter, simply because 2–0 = 122–120. In other words, the magnitude of the no-treatment profile, or the health prospect in the comparator, is neglected.

There are two principal reasons why the hidden parameter, E_{COMP}, matters in a priority-setting context: *caring* and *equality*. Caring means that the worse the health prospect without the intervention, the stronger our feeling of mercy and compassion, and, hence, the more duty we feel to provide intervention. The first Norwegian priority-setting guidelines (from 1987) had a strong emphasis on the *severity of illness* and suggested that this should be the primary concern when setting health care priorities. However, the revised guidelines (from 1997) took a broader perspective and include the importance of treatment effects and costs.

Focusing on the no-treatment profile resembles an understanding of 'need as ill health' as opposed to the health economic understanding of 'need as capacity to benefit' (see end of Chapter 4). Various attempts have been made in the literature to weight QALY gains depending on the severity of the illness, i.e. the worse the health prospect without treatment, the higher the weight assigned to the potential incremental health gains (see e.g. Nord, 1995).

The second reason why E_{COMP} matters relates to a concern for *equality in prospective health*. When comparing two patient groups, A and B, with different health prospects without treatment ($E_{COMP}^A < E_{COMP}^B$) but identical potential gains from treatment ($\Delta E^A = \Delta E^B$), inequalities in prospective health will be reduced if the group with the shortest prospective health is prioritized. Therefore, when E_{COMP} is small, we would accept a smaller ΔE, suggesting preferences for *equality in relative gains*: $\Delta E / E_{COMP}$.

15.4 Age: equality in total health

The no-treatment profile, E_{COMP}, and the incremental gains, ΔE, are two prospective streams of health, both of which can be identified within the ICER.

Table 15.1 Three patient groups with different combinations of health gains, no-treatment profiles, and age

Patient group	A	B	C
Streams of health			
Health gains	9	8	8
No-treatment profile	3	1	3
Distribution of *prospective health* if:			
A is prioritized	12	1	3
B is prioritized	3	9	3
C is prioritized	3	1	11
Age	60	60	30
Distribution of *total health* if:			
A is prioritized	72	61	33
B is prioritized	63	69	33
C is prioritized	63	61	41

When looking *retrospectively*, patient age emerges as a separate stream of health.[2] The importance of differences in age was introduced to the health economics literature by the late Alan Williams, himself a leading QALY-gain advocate who held that every individual deserves their 'fair innings' of health (Williams, 1997). The older the individual is and the better health they have experienced, the less they are entitled to more health, compared with people who have *not* had their 'fair innings' of health.

Table 15.1 provides a numerical example of three patients who are similar in every respect except for the QALY numbers associated with the three different streams of health, namely: health gains, no-treatment profile, and age. The exercise here is to prioritize *one* patient group on the basis of the partial information provided in each line and any previous ones, moving sequentially down the rows. In other words, prioritize first on the basis of the information about differences in health gains *only*, i.e. assume everything else is similar. Then move down and take into account the additional information about the differences in no-treatment profiles, and prioritize on the basis of this combined information about health gains and no-treatment profiles (assume the patients' ages are identical). Depending on who is then prioritized, the table

---

[2] Retrospective health can be subdivided into one stream that is the result of past interventions, i.e. retrospective health gains, and one stream that has come 'for free', i.e. without any health care (Dolan and Olsen, 2001).

includes the alternative distributions of *prospective health*. Finally, take account of the age differences, and prioritize one of the three patients on the basis of their differences in health gain, no-treatment profile *and* age. At the bottom, the table shows the alternative distributions of *total health*—depending on which of the three is prioritized.

If the only information that distinguishes the three patients were their prospective health gain (first row), we would probably prioritize A. Note that there is no trade-off involved. With the additional information on the no-treatment profile (second row), we notice a trade-off between maximizing health (i.e. opt for A) *or* reduce inequalities in prospective health (i.e. opt for B). There is no one correct answer here—it depends on your preferences vis-à-vis maximizing health or *reducing inequalities in prospective health*. But the likelihood is that we would opt for B. The degree of inequality in prospective health between top and bottom will be 3 (9 vs 3) if we prioritize B, as opposed to 12 (12 vs 1) if we prioritize A.

Then, with the additional information about the patients' ages (retrospective health), if we *reduce inequalities in total lifetime health* we are drawn from B towards C. This is where the degree of inequality in total health between top and bottom is lowest (63 vs 41). Note that the health gains are similar for B and C, so we are faced with a trade-off between severity and age. If we are concerned with equalities in *prospective* health, we would be drawn to B; if we are concerned with equalities in *total* health, we would be drawn towards C.

In general, there are various ways in which people's strength of preferences for equality in health can be elicited, regarding both their inequality aversion per se and which stream of health they think should be the primary focus of attention, i.e. whether they are concerned with reducing inequalities in prospective health or in total health.[3]

Beyond age, there is another retrospective health issue in the duration and magnitude of *past suffering*. Generally, we care more for people who have suffered a lot, which may explain why hospital waiting time is an issue that receives persistent policy attention. The opposite of past *suffering* is past *health gains*. Intuitively, this may seem an unexpected issue to bring into the priority debate. However, its potential relevance is likely to depend on the *cause* of the ill health that preceded the need for the health care which produced past health gains (Dolan and Olsen, 2001).

....

[3] See e.g. Dolan, T. and Tsuchiya, A. (2005) Health priorities and public preferences: the relative importance of past health experience and future health prospects. *Journal of Health Economics*, **24**, 703–14.

15.5 **Causes of ill health**

Going back to Part 2, Figure 5.1 illustrates the three major causes of ill health. First, *genetics* explains inherited diseases through natural variations in human biology. Second, the physical and social *environment* includes working conditions, pollution, cultural norms and position in the social hierarchy. Third, health-related *lifestyle* refers to people's behaviour regarding their diet, exercise, and substance use.

The reason why, in a priority-setting context, we are concerned with these three classes of health *determinants* is that they strike people differently. Inequalities in health arise because of inequalities—or variations—in how different groups of people are exposed to these determinants. Which types of inequalities would society consider *unjust* or *unfair*, to the extent that we introduce compensatory measures to reduce them?

First, nature—the biological lottery—is neither just nor unjust. It is not a normative issue that we can agree or disagree with. Still, we may agree or disagree with the extent to which society *should compensate* those who have been unlucky in this lottery. Note that the most frequently stated argument in favour of compensation is that people with inherited diseases are unfortunate in that they had no control over the cause of their illness—they are 'without fault of their own'.

While biological differences are unavoidable (at least in the short run), environmental differences are to a larger extent avoidable (at least if they are man made). The recent WHO commission on social determinants of health[4] was concerned with the extent to which an inequality is *avoidable*: 'The vast majority of inequalities in health, between and within countries, are avoidable and, hence, inequitable,' and 'No country or region should have to live with ill health that is avoidable.' Interestingly, most ill health in the world would be 'avoidable' had we spent more resources to prevent or to cure it. Pragmatically, this is an issue of costs vs effects. The question is why this notion of 'avoidability' in itself may have any normative power.

The concept is used in relation to 'social deprivation', and thereby reflects a view that society has a special duty to reduce inequalities in ill health that have a social cause. The policy concern of this issue can be seen in thick government reports and in political debates, as well as in media attention in many countries, e.g. the UK and Norway. The suggested methodological solution to how this objective of reduced social inequalities in health can be accounted for in

---

[4] http://www.who.int/social_determinants/en/

economic evaluations is to assign 'social class weights' to outcomes, so that a QALY gained among socially deprived patient groups has a weighting higher than unity.

Interestingly, while social causes of ill health might be avoidable through other social and economic policies, 'unhealthy lifestyles' would in principle be even more *avoidable* if people changed their behaviour. However, the concept of *responsibility* is being used at the individual level, i.e. the view that people should be held responsible for their own health-related behaviour.

Some economists and ethicists have focused on this notion of individual *responsibilities* for own health: if there is 'equity of choice', then those inequalities that may follow from differences in preferences (behaviour) are not considered inequitable.[5] And, if not inequitable, they are by logic equitable, i.e. we should not worry about inequalities in health that reflect differences in lifestyle. This involves a shift in health policy focus from *equal consequences* to *equal opportunities*. The fundamental problem, though, is the extent to which people *can* be held responsible, i.e. how much of an observed health-related lifestyle reflects genuine individual preferences and how much is social conditioning?

The strong correlation between *social deprivation* and *unhealthy lifestyles* suggests that there may be recursive effects between the two variables. This seems like a tricky health policy dilemma: on the one hand should society compensate for the social gradient by allocating *more* health care resources to the socially deprived, and on the other should unhealthy choices be discouraged because of their increased health care cost implications? But in a priority-setting context, it is perfectly consistent to apply two sets of health policy interventions. By levying indirect taxes (see Chapter 6) on unhealthy behaviour, consumers are faced with the full costs to society of their health-related choices, quite independently on their social position. This type of intervention deals with the social costs of health-related consumption. The second type of intervention deals with the social benefits associated with reduced deprivation.

15.6 **Consequences beyond patients' health gains**

Cost-effectiveness analyses usually measure and value health outcomes in the treated patients only. Beyond this, there are other sets of potential benefits. First, the direct 'health-to-health' externalities (Chapter 3) that should be

---

[5] See e.g. Le Grand, 1987, 1991; Devooght, 2004; Cappelen and Nordheim, 2005.

included as part of the aggregated health outcomes. Such externalities are important in poor countries where a significant slice of health care budgets is spent on combating communicable diseases.

A second set of health externalities is the positive impact on other household members' well-being, e.g. the impact on small children of their parents' improved health, and the impact on elderly relatives of improved health in those who care for them. Furthermore, when curing addiction and substance abuse, there is immense positive health-related impact in terms of relieved anxiety and misery among other members of the household, as well as the local community. When accounting for such positive externalities, this is not weighting individuals in accordance with their importance to other people. Rather, it is consistent with a utilitarian idea of aggregating all utility impacts in all affected individuals—not only the patients.

Beyond the impact on other people's health and well-being, there are potential economic contributions to society as measured in production gains (PG), the distributive implications of which have been discussed above. One aspect in the discussion on the inclusion of PG was the extent to which *future* contributions to the health sector would outweigh the cost of treatment. Interestingly, 'merit' as something that enhances an individual's entitlement to health care refers to *past* contributions, such as having made contributions to society or in other ways having proved to be a deserving citizen. In a priority-setting context, however, this 'merit' issue is one that belongs more to the individual level than the patient-group level.

15.7 Conclusion

The key priority-setting problem with cost benefit analyses—in a health policy setting guided by an objective of 'equal access for equal need, independent of income'—is simply its use of a benefit measure that depends on income. The priority-setting problems with cost-effectiveness analyses are that the ICER i) hides priority-relevant parameters *inside* its formulae, and ii) ignores issues that lie *outside* its formulae.

As a summary, Table 15.2 lists potentially priority-relevant issues discussed in this chapter and give examples of how they differ across two patients, A and B, both of whom stand to gain 1 QALY. The first column in the table lists the issues: severity (no-treatment profile), previous health (age, past illnesses), cause of current disease (inherited, social, lifestyle), consequences on others (well-being, economic contribution), and merit (past contributions). For each of these issues, you are asked to make a *partial* judgement of the described difference between A and B, and fill in the last column. Ignore any of the

Table 15.2 Examples of differences in some characteristics of potential relevance in health care priority setting

	A 1 QALY gain	B 1 QALY gain	A, B, or indifferent?
No-treatment profile	1 year in ill health	10 healthy years	
Age	75	25	
Past illnesses (without own fault)	5 years' suffering	No past illnesses	
Inherited disease	Yes	No	
Social class	Deprived	Affluent	
Influenced by unhealthy lifestyle	Yes	No	
Consequences on others' well-being	None	Positive impacts	
Economic contribution to society	None	Large	
Past contributions to society	Large	None	

other differences, and consider the extent to which the partial information *alone* would make you prioritize A or B (remember their potential gain is the same).

If you are indifferent in *every* choice in Table 15.2, you appear to be a pure QALY maximizer. If not, you are prepared to make trade-offs between health gains and the other listed characteristic(s). If you have strong preferences for either A or B in one or more of the described differences, you may increase or decrease the QALY gain for either A or B until you end up with no difference. You are then faced with your own trade-off between efficiency (as total QALY maximization), and your preference for the other characteristic.

It is certainly possible in principle to elicit people's trade-offs on the above issues, and many recent studies have attempted to do so. However, different approaches have yielded some very different magnitudes in the implicit weights, and have created controversy in the literature. While the literature is waiting for more convincing quantitative weights that health economists and policy makers may agree on, I would suggest that an economic evaluation should include a systematic qualitative description of the implication of a health care programme on other priority-relevant variables. For this purpose, an 'equity checklist' can be developed, as in Box 15.1.

A checklist of equity issues

1. What is the *size of the health gain* to the average patient: negligible or significant?

2. What is the *severity*, i.e. what will happen without (or with the existing) treatment? What is the remaining life-expectancy in the comparator? What is the expected health state in the comparator?

3. How much *past health* have the patients already had? Which age group? How much ill health have they had, and for how long?

4. Are there any *'causal characteristics'* with the patients or the illness? Any inherited diseases? Any social deprivation or other environmental exposure? Any health-related behaviour?

5. Are there any *wider consequences* beyond the treated patients' improved health? Will there be any impact on the health or well-being of other household members? Will there be an economic contribution to the rest of society?

Suggested reading

Williams, A. (1997) Intergenerational equity: an exploration of the 'fair innings' argument. *Health Economics*, 6, 117–32.

Olsen, J. A., Richardson, J., Dolan, P. and Menzel, P. (2003) The moral relevance of personal characteristics in setting health care priorities. *Social Science and Medicine*, 57, 1163–172.

Mason, H., Jones-Lee, M. and Donaldson, C. (2008) Modelling the monetary value of a QALY: a new approach based on UK data. *Health Economics*.

Exercises

1. Do you agree that 'a QALY is a QALY is a QALY'? If not, based on the issues listed in the first column of Table 15.2, when do you think a QALY is *not* a QALY is *not* a QALY?

2. Imagine you are a health care decision maker presented with the ICER figure for the new treatment programme. You are then allowed to ask for information about three additional issues (including those listed in Table 15.2). Which would be most important to you? Explain.

3. Final exercise: continue studying health economics and policy with an open—and critical—mind!

References

Beattie, J., Covey, J., Dolan, P., Hopkins, L., Jones-Lee, M., Loomes, G., Pidgeon, N., Robinson, A. and Spencer, A. (1998) On the contingent valuation of safety and the safety of contingent valuation: part 1—caveat investigator. *Journal of Risk and Uncertainty*, 17, 5–25.

Biørn, E., Hagen, T. P., Iversen, T. and Magnussen, J. (2003) The effects of activity-based hospital efficiency: A panel data analysis of DEA efficiency scores 1992–2000. *Health Care Management Science*, 6, 271–83.

Cairns, J. A. and van der Pol, M. M (1997) Constant and decreasing timing aversion. *Social Science and Medicine*, 45 (11), 1653–9.

Cappelen, A. W. and Nordheim, O. F. (2005) Responsibility in health care: a liberal egalitarian approach. *Journal of Medical Ethics*, 31, 476–80.

Clark, D. and Olsen, J. A. (1994) Agency in health care with an endogenous budget constraint. *Journal of Health Economics*, 13, 231–51.

Culyer, A. J. (1989) The normative economics of health care finance and provision. *Oxford Review of Economic Policy*, 5 (1), 34–58.

Culyer, A. J. (2001) Equity—some theory and its policy implications. *Journal of Medical Ethics*, 27, 275–83.

Daniels, N. (1985) *Just Health Care*. Cambridge: Cambridge University Press.

Devooght, K. (2004) On responsibility-sensitive egalitarian ethics. *Ethics and Economics*, 2 (2), 1–21.

Dolan, P. and Olsen, J. A. (2001) Equity in health: the importance of different health streams. *Journal of Health Economics*, 20, 823–34.

Dolan, T. and Tsuchiya, A. (2005) Health priorities and public preferences: the relative importance of past health experience and future health prospects. *Journal of Health Economics*, 24, 703–14.

Drummond, M. F., Sculpher, M. J., Torrance, G. W., O'Brien, B. J. and Stoddart, G. L. (2005) *Methods for the Economic Evaluation of Health Care Programmes*. Oxford: Oxford University Press.

Elster, J. (1992) *Local justice: how institutions allocate scarce goods and necessary burdens*. New York: Russell Sage.

Evans, R. G. (1984) *Strained Mercy: The economics of Canadian health care*. Toronto: Butterworths.

Evans, R. G., Barer, M. and Marmor, T. (ed.) (1994) *Why are some people healthy and others not? The determinants of health of populations*. New York: Gruyter.

Fox-Rushby, J. and Cairns, J. (2005) *Economic Evaluation*. Maidenhead: Open University Press.

Fuchs, V. (1986) Physician-induced demand: A parable. *Journal of Health Economics*, 5, 367.

Gottret, P. and Schieber, G. (2006) *Health financing revisited: A practitioner's guide*. Washington DC: The World Bank.

Grossmann, M. (1972) On the concept of health capital and the demand for health. *Journal of Political Economy*, 80, 223–55.

Hagen, T. P. and Kaarbøe, O. M. (2006) The Norwegian hospital reform of 2002: Central government takes over ownership of public hospitals. *Health Policy*, 76, 320–33.

Harsanyi, J. (1955) Cardinal welfare, individualistic ethics and interpersonal comparisons of utility. *Journal of Political Economy*, 63, 309–21.

Harsanyi, J. (1975) Can the maximin principle serve as a basis for morality? A critique of John Rawls's theory. *American Political Science Review*, 69, 594–606.

Iversen, T. (2005) A study of income-motivated behaviour among general practitioners in the Norwegian list patient system. *HERO Working Paper 2005:8* (Health Economics Research Programme at University of Oslo).

Iversen, T. and Lurås, H. (2006) Capitation and incentives in primary care. In *The Elgar Companion to Health Economics* (ed. A. Jones). Cheltenham: E. Elgar Publishing.

Jegers, M., Kesteloot, K., De Graeve, D. and Gilles, W. (2002) A typology for provider payment systems in health care. *Health Policy*, 60 (3), 255–73.

Le Grand, J. (1991) *Equity and choice*. London: Harper Collins.

Le Grand, J. (1987) Equity, health and health care. *Social Justice Research*, 1, 257–74.

Magnussen, J., Hagen, T. P. and Kaarbø, O. (2007) Centralized or decentralized? A case study of Norwegian hospital reform. *Social Science & Medicine*, 64, 2129–37.

Manning, W. G., Newhouse, J. P., Duan, N. *et al.* (1987) Health Insurance and the demand for medical care: Evidence from a randomized experiment. *The American Economic Review*, 77 (3), 251–77.

Mannion, R. and Davies, H. T. O. (2008) Payment for performance in health care. *British Medical Journal*, 336, 306–08.

Marmot, M. (2004) *The status syndrome: How social standing affects our health and longevity*. New York: Times Books.

Morris, S., Devlin, N. and Parkin, D. (2007) *Economic analysis in health care*. Chichester: John Wiley.

Neuhauser, D. and Lewicki, A. M. (1975) What do we gain from the sixth stool guiac? *New England Journal of Medicine*, 293 (5), 226–8.

Nord, E. (1995) The person-trade-off approach to valuing health care programmes. *Medical Decision Making*, 15 (3), 201–8.

Olsen, J. A. (1997) Theories of justice and their implications for priority setting in health care. *Journal of Health Economics*, 16, 625–40.

Olsen, J. A. and Richardson, J. (1999) Production gains from health care: What should be included in cost-effectiveness analyses? *Social Science and Medicine*, 49, 17–26.

Olsen, J. A., Donaldson, C. and Pereira, J. (2004) The insensitivity of 'willingness to pay' to the size of the good: new evidence for health care. *Journal of Economic Psychology*, 25, 445–60.

Pennant-Rea, R. and Emmott, W. (1983) *The Pocket Economist*. Oxford: Basil Blackwell.

Rawls, J. (1971) *A Theory of Justice*, Cambridge MA: Harvard University Press.

Reinhardt, U. E. (1998) Abstracting from distributional effects, this policy is effective. In *Health, health care and health economics: Perspectives on distribution* (ed. M. L. Barer, T. E. Getzen and G. L. Stoddart). Chichester: John Wiley.

Rice, D. and Cooper, B. (1967) The economic value of human life. *American Journal of Public Health*, 57, 1954–66.

Skrabanek, P. (1994) *The death of humane medicine and the rise of coercive healthism.* Suffolk: Crowley Esmonde.

Thaler, R. H. and Sunstein, C. R. (2008) *Nudge: improving decisions about health, wealth, and happiness.* New Haven: Yale University Press.

Tengs, T. O., Adams, M. E., Pliskin, J. S. *et al.* (1995) Five hundred life-saving interventions and their cost effectiveness. *Risk Analysis*, 15 (3), 369–90.

Varian, H. (1975) Distributive justice, welfare economics, and the theory of fairness. *Philosophy and Public Affairs*, 4, 223–47.

Wagstaff, A. (2007) Social health insurance re-examined. WPS 4111. Washington DC: The World Bank (available at www.worldbank.org).

Weinstein, M. C., Siegel, J. E., Garber, A. M., Lipscombe, J., Luce, B. R., Manning, W. G. and Torrance, G. W. (1997) Productivity costs, time costs and health-related quality of life: A response to the Erasmus Group. *Health Economics*, 6, 505–10.

Wilkinson, R. G. (1996) *Unhealthy societies: the affliction of inequality.* London: Routledge.

Williams, A. (1988) Ethics and efficiency in the provision of health care. In *Philosophy and medical welfare* (ed. J. M. Bell and S. Mendus). Cambridge: Cambridge University Press.

Williams, A. (1997) Intergenerational equity: An exploration of the 'fair innings' argument. *Health Economics*, 6, 117–32.

Williams, A. and Cookson, R. (2000) Equity in health. In *Handbook of Health Economics* (ed. A. J. Culyer and J. P. Newhouse). Amsterdam: Elsevier.

Index

actuarially fair insurance 113–15
adverse selection 114–15
agency relationship 52–5
allocative efficiency 157–8
altruism 62–7
asymmetric information 52–5

benefits forgone 35, 36, 71, 76
budget line 25–8, 32, 43, 46
burden of disease 183

capitation 139, 143–5
'caring externality' 52
compulsary public insurance 119–24
contagion 56–8
cost–benefit analysis (CBA) 170, 186, 201, 208
cost-effectiveness analysis (CEA) 171, 208, 214
cost–utility analysis (CUA) 171
costs
    average 196–8
    marginal 196–8
    production losses 200
    technical optimum 197
cream skimming 57
cross-subsidy 58, 106, 114, 116

deductibles
    insurance plans 129–31, 134
demand curve 39, 40, 41, 42, 57, 86–8, 112,
    130, 141, 142
demand, elasticities of 40–2
determinants of health 83
diagnosis-related group (DRG) 156, 157, 200
diet 95, 96–7, 213
disability-adjusted life year (DALY) 182–4
discounting 201–4
distributive justice, theories of 67–72
doctor–patient relationship 52–4

economic evaluation 169–74, 187, 201–4, 213
efficiency
    allocative 44
    cost 25–6, 43
    technical 25, 43
egalitarianism 69
environment
    see physical environment
    and social environment
EQ-5D descriptive instrument 4, 180
equality 78–9
equity 79

externalities 50–9, 61, 86–8
'fair innings' of age 211
fairness 80
fee for service 149–51

genetics 83, 213

health
    descriptive systems 3–6, 14–15
    dimensions of 5
health care
    definition of 6, 15
health possibility frontier (HPF)
    defined 37–8
    social welfare function 75–7
    theories of justice and 72–5
health gains
    consequences beyond patients' 214–15
    generally 209–10
    monetary value of 189–92
health-related lifestyle
    interventions 101
    substance use 95, 98–101
health-related quality of life (HRQL) 4,
    178, 179
health span 5, 6, 95, 189
healthy life expectancy (HALE) 5
human capital 58, 207

incremental cost-effective ratio (ICER) 192,
    193, 210
indifference curve 29–30, 31
individual preferences 92, 192, 214
inequalities, health care 15, 78, 79, 89, 90, 92
insurance
    see compulsory public insurance
    and voluntary insurance
internal markets 138, 163, 165–6
isocost see budget line
isoquant 24–6

justice 80–1

labour supply 122, 145–8
life expectancy 11–14, 91

marginal costs 39, 42, 51, 86, 87, 112, 131–2,
    143, 165, 195–8
marginal productivity 21, 38, 73, 198
marginal utility 23, 30, 62, 68, 108, 202
maximin 70–2

monetary benefits 175, 192
monopoly 47, 51
moral hazard 112–13, 127

national health service (NHS) 121–2, 151, 153
needs 9, 17, 53, 68, 70, 133, 142
non-welfarist 66, 209

opportunity costs 35–6, 38, 76, 77, 146, 165

Pareto
efficient 34, 38, 43–4
improvement 34
optimal 36
potential Pareto criterion 172
patient payment
co-payment 128–9, 134, 135
distributive implications 131–2
perfect competition 19, 186
perfect market model 47–52
physical environment
externalities 88
generally 85–9
pollution 85
polluter pay principle 86–7
prevention 6, 7, 8, 15
primary goods 69, 70–1, 78
priority setting 169–74, 210, 215
private insurance see voluntary insurance
private goods 48, 49, 50
production functions 19–22, 53
production gains 73, 170, 176, 185–8, 193,
199, 207
production losses 186, 199
production possibility frontier (PPF) 33, 34,
37, 43
productivity 21, 22, 24
provider remuneration
primary care
capitation see capitation
fee for service see fee for service
salary see salary
secondary care
hospital payment systems 154–9
public bad 85–6
public goods 49, 50, 55, 58, 65, 86, 188

quality-adjusted life years (QALYs) 6, 73,
176, 178–82, 192, 193, 216
quality of life 4, 172, 178–81

redistribution 62–4
income 90
regulation
direct 88, 99, 100
indirect 88
rehabilitation 6, 7, 8, 15, 164, 165, 200
revenue–expenditure–income identity 103,
106, 137, 166

risk behaviour 107–8, 116
risk pooling 107

salary
capitation compared 149–51
fee for service compared 149–51
generally 145–8
smoking 50, 96, 102
social environment
education and 89
health and 89, 90
income distribution 89–90
inequalities in health 89, 92
social hierarchy 90–1
social health insurance 120–4
social welfare function (SWF) 75–7, 209
split preferences 55
standard gamble 180–2
substance use 98–101
substitution 26–32
supply curve 39, 40, 42, 86, 141
supply, demand and 37–44

target income hypothesis 143, 148
taxed-financed insurance 121–4
technical efficiency 25, 43, 51, 156
time preference rate 201
trade offs
consumers and 30
health/wealth 31
income/leisure 147, 200
person 182
time 180
transaction costs 115, 116, 150, 165
transfer payments 185
transfers in cash 64–7
transfers in-kind 64–7
transformation curve see production
possibility frontier

uncertainty 49, 52, 71, 107, 165, 174, 182, 202
utilitarianism 67–9, 77–8
utility functions 22–3
utility possibility frontier (UPF) 36, 37, 77

visual analogue scale 180–182
voluntary donations 58, 61, 103
voluntary insurance
actuarially fair insurance 113–15
adverse selection 114–16
compulsory public insurance
compared 123
moral hazard 112–13

wealth
health and 9, 10, 30–1
welfarist 66, 209
willingness-to-pay (WTP) 190–2, 201, 207–8